The Essential HRT Primer

The Essential HRT Primer

Editors:
Murray Fingeret, OD
John G. Flanagan, PhD, MCOptom
Jeffrey M. Liebmann, MD

Contributing Authors:
Alfonso Antón, MD
Balwantray C. Chauhan, PhD
George A. Cioffi, MD
David F. Garway-Heath, MD, FRCOphth
Christopher A. Girkin, MD
Chris Hudson, PhD
Chris A. Johnson, PhD
Robert N. Weinreb, MD
Linda M. Zangwill, PhD

Jocoto Advertising, Inc.
San Ramon, California

Jocoto Advertising, Inc., San Ramon 94583
© 2005 by Heidelberg Engineering
All rights reserved. Published 2005
Printed in the United States of America
14 13 12 11 10 09 08 07 06 05   1 2 3 4 5

ISBN (cloth): 0-976875608
            978-0-9768756-0-4

EAN: 9780976875604

This book is printed on acid-free paper.

About the Authors

Murray Fingeret, OD
Chief, Optometry Section
Veterans Administration,
New York Harbor Health Care System
Clinical Professor, State University of New York
College of Optometry, New York, NY

Jeffrey M. Liebmann, MD
Clinical Professor of Ophthalmology, Director,
Glaucoma Services, Manhattan Eye, Ear &
Throat Hospital and New York University
Medical Center, New York, NY

John G. Flanagan, PhD, MCOptom
Professor, School of Optometry,
University of Waterloo, Waterloo;
Professor, Department of Ophthalmology
and Vision Sciences,
University of Toronto, Toronto;
Senior Scientist, Vision Science Research
Program, & Director, Glaucoma Research Unit,
Toronto Western Hospital Research Institute,
University Health Network, Toronto,
Ontario, Canada

Alfonso Antón, MD
Chief of Glaucoma
Instituto de Oftalmobiología
Aplicada (IOBA)
Universidad de Valladolid
Glaucoma Service
Hospital de la Esperanza y el Mar
Instituto Municipal de Asistencia Sanitaria
(IMAS), Barcelona, Spain

Balwantray C. Chauhan, PhD
Professor, Research Director,
and Chair in Vision Research
Department of Ophthalmology
Dalhousie University
Halifax, Nova Scotia, Canada

George A. Cioffi, MD
Chief, Ophthalmology
Director, Glaucoma Service
Devers Eye Institute
Legacy Health System
Portland, Oregon

David F. Garway-Heath, MD, FRCOphth
Clinical Research Lead,
Glaucoma Research Unit
Moorfields Eye Hospital
London, England

Christopher A. Girkin, MD
Associate Professor of Ophthalmology
Director, Glaucoma Service
University of Alabama at Birmingham
Birmingham, Alabama

Chris Hudson, PhD
Associate Professor, School of Optometry,
University of Waterloo, Waterloo;
Associate Professor, Department of
Ophthalmology and Vision Sciences,
University of Toronto, Toronto, Ontario, Canada

Chris A. Johnson, PhD
Director of Diagnostic Research
Discoveries in Sight
Devers Eye Institute
Portland, Oregon

Robert N. Weinreb, MD
Distinguished Professor Of Ophthalmology
Director, Hamilton Glaucoma Center
Professor, University of California, San Diego
La Jolla, California

Linda M. Zangwill, PhD
Director, Diagnostic Imaging Laboratory,
Hamilton Glaucoma Center
Professor, Department of Ophthalmology
University of California, San Diego
La Jolla, California

Contents

	Foreword *Robert N. Weinreb*	
Chapter 1	Principles of Confocal Scanning Laser Ophthalmoscopy for the Clinician *Christopher A. Girkin*	1
Chapter 2	Using the Heidelberg Retina Tomograph II (HRT II): Image Acquisition and Accessing the Data *Murray Fingeret*	11
Chapter 3	Moorfields Regression Analysis *David F. Garway-Heath*	31
Chapter 4	Clinical Interpretation of the Heidelberg Retina Tomograph II (HRT II) *Alfonso Antón*	41
Chapter 5	Detection of Glaucomatous Changes in the Optic Disc *Balwantray C. Chauhan*	53
Chapter 6	Structural/Functional Relationships in Glaucoma *George A. Cioffi and Chris A. Johnson*	67
Chapter 7	The Retina Module *John G. Flanagan and Chris Hudson*	77
Chapter 8	Use of the Heidelberg Retina Tomograph (HRT) in the Ocular Hypertension Treatment Study (OHTS) *Linda M. Zangwill and Robert N. Weinreb*	85
Chapter 9	The Importance of Optic Nerve Imaging in Clinical Practice *Jeffrey M. Liebmann*	91
	HRT Primer Cases *Murray Fingeret*	95
	Suggested Readings	121

FOREWORD
Robert N. Weinreb, MD

Glaucoma is a progressive optic neuropathy, and it makes sense that the examination of the optic nerve should be at the core of glaucoma testing for diagnosis and follow-up. However, this was considerably different 25 years ago. Prevailing dogma at that time recognized a triad of glaucomatous signs including characteristic visual field loss with manual kinetic perimetry, an enlarged "cup" of the glaucomatous optic disc, and high intraocular pressure. Standard static threshold automated perimetry was on the verge of being introduced into clinical practice. The optic disc was examined largely with the monocular view of the direct ophthalmoscope or an occasional stereoscopic glimpse with a separate lens.

For most practitioners, primary open-angle glaucoma was still conceptualized as a disease of high intraocular pressure and the clinical examination emphasized the office measurement of intraocular pressure and, occasionally, diurnal pressure testing. The level of intraocular pressure determined whether treatment would be initiated (or advanced, as appropriate). Ocular hypertensive patients with normal-appearing visual fields and optic discs were treated by lowering IOP to below 21 mm Hg. Glaucoma patients also were treated by lowering IOP to below 21 mm Hg, regardless of the stage of the disease.

In the late 1970s and early into the next decade, glaucoma diagnosis and management began to change. Automated visual field testing was quickly adopted in the early 1980s, and offered the clinician a standardized office test with improved reproducibility that did not depend on the availability of a highly skilled visual field technician. A few of us thought that the evaluation of the optic disc also could be improved by making it objective, quantitative, reproducible, rapid and, most of all, practical.

Very few ideas in medicine or biology ever prove to be entirely original, however. Concepts that seem original are almost always derived from earlier work. And, in this case, there had been unsuccessful attempts made to develop and implement quantitative disc assessment into clinical practice. Although there were existing quantitative methods for analyzing optic disc photographs, and other specialized imaging systems were soon to be developed that each had enthusiasts and supporters, these attempts stalled as they were laborious, required widely dilated pupils and clear media, or required hardware or software that was too expensive. This was about to change.

In early 1984, it seemed reasonable to employ a confocal imaging system to evaluate the optic disc. For those few of us in La Jolla, California and Heidelberg, Germany who had the opportunity to contribute to the conceptualization and testing of the first confocal scanning laser ophthalmoscope to assess optic disc topography, there was unbridled optimism. We were convinced that clinicians everywhere would be able to take advantage of the substantial benefits of optic disc imaging with the confocal laser ophthalmoscope to better diagnose and follow glaucoma.

Progress in medicine is often slow, however. In many circumstances, it is insufficient to merely have a better method. As I learned, a novel idea can be so far ahead of its time that contemporaries do not uniformly understand it. During the development period, manuscript reviews were often harsh and bewildering. Grant reviews even questioned the feasibility of the technology, and whether it could ever be implemented. I also learned that the introduction and adoption into clinical practice of a new idea depends on communication, cooperation, and collaboration to take it past the point where there is an imperative for change that is manifest, surging and, even, unstoppable.

Despite countless obstacles, some of us persisted in developing and working with the new technology. In the late 1980s, the first commercial confocal scanning laser ophthalmoscope (Laser Tomographic Scanner: Heidelberg Instruments) was built and tested. By 1991, the instrument was improved considerably (Heidelberg Retina Tomograph [HRT]: Heidelberg Engineering) and it was sufficiently reliable, effective, and convenient to implement into clinical practice. Academic glaucoma specialists, in particular, began using it for some clinical decisions. Nevertheless, it was not until reimbursement within the United States was obtained in 1999 that the confocal scanning laser ophthalmoscope gained widespread acceptance. By that time, there were hundreds of published manuscripts that tested and validated the technology. Clinicians now had, for the first time, an unsurpassed tool for objectively assessing optic disc topography, and they embraced it with enthusiasm.

Today, the central importance of the optic nerve in glaucoma is generally accepted. It is recognized that the optic disc examination is at the diagnostic core for recognizing glaucoma and detecting progression. Approximately two decades after testing the first prototype of a confocal scanning laser ophthalmoscope for optic disc assessment, this instrument is used in clinicians' offices throughout the world. The subjectivity of optic disc assessment has largely been removed. The communication, cooperation, and collaboration that led to the development of the instrument has escalated. Paraphrasing the conclusions of a November 2003 AIGS global consensus meeting on glaucoma diagnosis held in San Diego:[1] a method for detecting abnormality and documenting optic nerve structure should be part of routine clinical management of glaucoma; the sensitivity and specificity of imaging instruments are comparable to that of expert interpretation of stereo color photographs; and digital imaging, including the use of the confocal scanning laser ophthalmoscope, is recommended as a clinical tool to augment the assessment of the optic disc in the management of glaucoma.

Despite this sanguine view of optic disc assessment with the confocal scanning laser ophthalmoscope, there is still much to do to improve it. Methods for reducing operator input (for example, to automate disc margin placement or eliminate it) are being evaluated. Methods to enhance algorithms that distinguish the glaucomatous optic disc from the nonglaucomatous disc also are being examined. Finally, assessment of progression is just beginning to be understood, and the imminent availability of data analysis from 10 years of longitudinal study with the confocal scanning laser ophthalmoscope offers the promise of definitive algorithms for monitoring progression. In other words, we all should recognize that where we stand today "… is not the end. It is not even the beginning of the end. But it is, perhaps, the end of the beginning" (Winston Churchill).

Robert N. Weinreb, MD
Hamilton Glaucoma Center
University of California, San Diego
La Jolla, California, USA

REFERENCE

1. Weinreb RN, Greve EL. *Glaucoma Diagnosis: Structure and Function*. The Hague: Kugler Publications; 2004:155-156.

1 Principles of Confocal Scanning Laser Ophthalmoscopy for the Clinician

Christopher A. Girkin, MD

THE EVOLUTION OF THE OPTIC DISC EXAMINATION

The examination of the optic disc is unique in many respects in that it provides an opportunity to directly observe the effects of progressive neurodegenerative diseases such as glaucoma on a microscopic scale. Since the advent of the direct ophthalmoscope, methods to develop better quantitative parameters that describe optic disc structure have been sought. Subjective estimation of the cup/disc area ratio has long been used to quantify the degree of cupping in glaucoma in the clinical setting. However, detection of progressive glaucomatous change in the optic disc using this method is extremely difficult, if not impossible, due to poor reproducibility and high inter- and intra-observer variability. This certainly is not surprising given the complex architecture of the optic disc and the difficulties associated with clinical examination. Attempting to reduce the subtleties of optic disc contour to a single linear variable, such as cup/disc ratio, is clearly inadequate and ignores much of the three-dimensional shape of the neuroretinal rim and optic cup.

Photography of the optic disc by monocular and stereophotographic techniques has been the traditional method to document the appearance and demonstrate longitudinal changes in the disc. However, these nonquantitative methods require subjective physician interpretation and can be difficult and time-consuming in a busy clinical practice. Over the past 20 years, more objective ocular imaging techniques have been developed in an effort to provide accurate, reproducible quantitative measurements of the contour of the optic disc.

The goal of this evolving process has been to develop a technique capable of obtaining reproducible topographic information that can provide a more objective method to detect characteristics of the optic disc indicative of glaucomatous optic neuropathy, and detect the changes over time in the shape of the optic disc associated with progressive glaucomatous damage. The culmination of these efforts has resulted in the development of confocal scanning laser ophthalmoscopy, which provides rapid, noninvasive, noncontact imaging of the ocular fundus. Unlike conventional photography, which obtains two-dimensional imaging, scanning laser techniques utilize confocal imaging methods to obtain high-resolution images both perpendicular (x-axis, y-axis) to optic axis and along the optic axis (z-axis) (Figure 1.1). Confocal imaging procedures were initially developed over 30 years ago as a technique to provide optical sectioning of biologic and industrial specimens. These principles have been subsequently modified for a variety of uses in ophthalmology including in-vivo corneal, retinal, and optic disc imaging.

The Heidelberg Retina Tomograph II (HRT II) represents the latest iteration in the application of confocal scanning laser ophthalmoscopy to the examination of the optic disc. The HRT II is a scanning laser ophthalmoscope specifically designed to acquire three-dimensional images of the optic nerve head and posterior pole. This instrument provides rapid, reproducible topographic measurements of the optic disc including the size of the optic disc, the contour and shape of the optic disc, neuroretinal rim, and optic cup, along with measurements of the peripapillary retina and nerve fiber layer. In addition, the HRT II is much easier to use in a clinical setting than its predecessor, the original Heidelberg Retina Tomograph (HRT). This newer instrument is much more compact, provides greater automation of image acquisition, standardizes many of the important aspects of the imaging process, and includes software capable of providing clinically valuable automated analysis not seen in prior versions.

PRINCIPLES OF OPERATION

Confocal scanning laser ophthalmoscopy

Both the HRT and HRT II utilize a rapid scanning 670-nm diode laser to acquire images of the posterior segment. The emitted beam is redirected in the x-axis and y-axis along a plane of focus perpendicular to the optic axis (z-axis) using two oscillating mirrors to obtain a 15° x 15°, two-dimensional image reflected from the surface of the retina and optic disc. A luminance detector measures the light reflected from each point in the image after passing through a confocal imaging aperture. The confocal aperture limits the depth from which reflected light reaches the detector to a narrow range centered around the location of a set focal plane on the retinal or optic disc surface. Light that is deeper or shallower than this focal plane (i.e., not in the specific focal plane) is suppressed to provide an optical section of the posterior pole corresponding to this set focal plane (Figure 1.1). The depth of the focal plane is automatically adjusted by shifting the confocal aperture to acquire multiple optical sections through

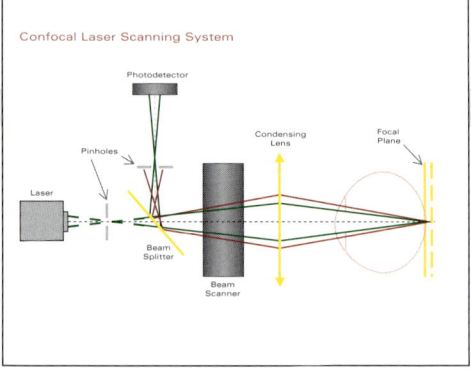

Figure 1.1

Schematic diagram of a confocal scanning laser system used in the HRT II.

the tissue of interest in order to create a layered three-dimensional image. Thus, the three-dimensional image contains information from multiple focal planes as the focal plane is shifted through the tissue — in this case, the optic disc.

The HRT II acquires reflectance images using 16 to 64 imaging planes to a depth of 4 mm. The number of optic sections increases at greater scan depth in order to image deeper optic cups. These optic sections are then combined to develop a three-dimensional contour map of the optic disc surface. The value of reflectance obtained from each focal plane at every point in the 15° image in the z-axis forms the z-profile for that point, from which a measurement of retinal height can be obtained from the distribution of the amount of reflected light along this z-axis. Thus, the z-profile of each point may be presented as a plot of reflectance intensity versus scan depth (Figure 1.2 A,B). The peak intensity from the z-profile plot is assumed to correspond to the location of internal limiting membrane that overlies the retina and optic disc (the internal limiting membrane of Elshnig). The final result produces a topographic map of 384 x 384 height measurements of retinal and/or optic disc surface topography.

THE HRT AND THE HRT II

The first commercially available instrument was the Heidelberg Retinal Tomograph (HRT), which was used primarily for clinical research. This confocal scanning laser has demonstrated excellent reproducibility, high sensitivity and specificity for the detection of glaucoma, and has provided very promising results with respect to the detection of progressive glaucomatous damage. In addition, this technology has been evaluated to a much greater extent than any existing optic disc or nerve fiber layer imaging system and is the device used in the confocal scanning laser ophthalmoscopy study performed as an ancillary project of the Ocular Hypertension Treatment Study (OHTS).[1,2] However, the HRT requires an experienced operator and fine-tuning of several manual settings in order to obtain high-quality images, which makes routine use of the

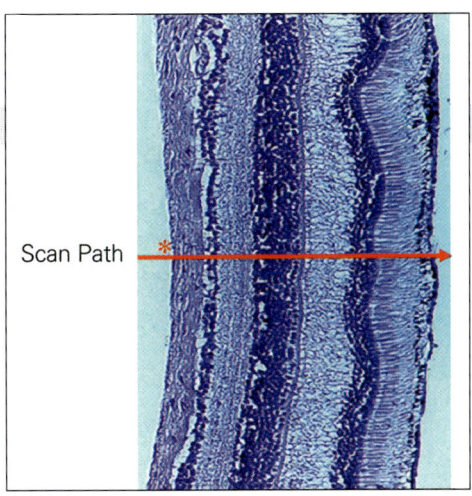

Figure 1.2A

The z-axis of the scan path (red arrow) of the scanning laser through the retina.

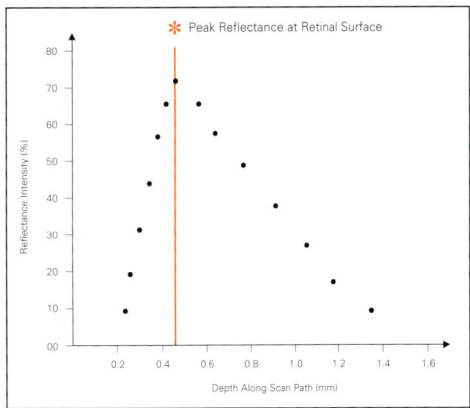

Figure 1.2B

Plot of reflectance intensity along this scan path for one point in the 384 X 384 pixel HRT II image. The peak reflectance along the z-axis is considered to correspond to the height of the retina surface (red asterisk) at that point.

HRT in the clinical setting difficult. The extensive experience gained from the development of the HRT along with ample clinical research using this instrument has provided the means to develop the more user-friendly HRT II.

The HRT II also utilizes a diode laser to acquire reflectance images. The theoretical resolution of both the HRT and the HRT II is similar and limited by the optics of the eye to 10 µm in transverse resolution and 300 µm in axial resolution (full width at half height). Peak-to-peak resolution in the axial plane is considerably less at approximately 50 to 60 µm. The much more compact HRT II has incorporated several automated scan procedures that have improved the ease of routine clinical use compared with prior versions of the HRT, which were considerably more cumbersome. These modifications include a higher resolution for the 15° image (the same as that used on the 10° scan of the HRT), a pre-scan planning mode, automatic selection of the fine focus and scan depth, automated serial scanning with built-in quality control measures, and automated averaging of serial scans.

The original HRT was able to obtain scans using three field size settings: 10° × 10°, 15° × 15°, or 20° × 20° centered on the optic disc. The resolution at any of these settings was 256 × 256 pixels. Thus, pixel size for the HRT varies from 10 to 26 µm per pixel depending on the scan area used. The HRT II in contrast is set to measure a 15° scan area. This change further automates the imaging process, provides a larger field of view to aid in centration of the optic disc and assessment of the nerve fiber layer, and minimizes vignetting of the optic disc at the edge of the scan field. In order to obtain a similar transverse resolution with the HRT II that is comparable to the maximal transverse resolution of the original HRT for a 10° image, the HRT II uses a higher resolution of 384 × 384 pixels. The higher number of pixels for the set 15° image maintains the highest resolution with the HRT II of 10 µm/pixel (the best resolution obtained using the 10° scanning field with the original HRT), making it possible to combine images from the two instruments for serial analysis (see Chapter 5).

With prior versions of the HRT, the fine focus and scan depth had to be adjusted manually. This process has been fully automated with the HRT II. Once the patient is positioned and the optic disc is in focus, the HRT II automatically performs a pre-scan through the optic disc when the unit is activated for imaging to determine the depth of the individual's optic nerve. This scan traverses through the optic disc. Using information from this pre-scan, the fine focus and scan depth are automatically adjusted to ensure that the entire optic disc is included on the imaging cross-sections.

Next, the HRT II uses this planning pre-scan to determine the number of imaging planes (planes of focus) to use that will incorporate the entire disc from the retinal surface to the base of the optic cup. The longitudinal field of view (the range of scan depth) of the current instrument ranges from 1 to 4 mm. Each successive scan plane is set to measure 0.0625 mm deeper as the scans are taken incrementally through the tissue. Thus, if the pre-scan determines that a 1 mm scan depth is required, 16 imaging planes will be used, whereas, if the depth is 4 mm, the imaging planes are increased to 64. Unlike the original HRT, in which the longitudinal resolution varies with scan depth, the HRT II maintains the axial resolution of the scan at 62 μm by varying the number of imaging planes. Thus, the HRT II maintains a constant digital resolution in both the transverse axis and longitudinal axis despite individual differences in the depth or size of the optic disc.

Finally, as mentioned previously, the HRT II automatically obtains three scans after the pre-scan for use in analysis. Automated quality control measures detect scans that are inadequate due to blinking and/or fixation shifts, and repeats the faulty scan to ensure that three adequate scans are obtained during each imaging session for analysis. The HRT II then automatically aligns and averages the scans to create the mean topography image for the scan session. This, more than any other feature of the HRT II, provides the foundation for its successful clinical application. It enables an individual assessment of the noise or variability of the images for a given eye at a given visit, therefore enabling the individually tailored analysis of progression. Many of these procedures had to be manually performed using the original HRT, adding to the difficulty in post-acquisition image processing.

PATIENT SAFETY

The 670-nm diode laser used in both the HRT and HRT II does not pose any safety hazard and is categorized as a Class 1 laser system. The intensity of the scanning diode laser is 100 times lower than the luminance of a digital fundus flash camera, making the imaging process much more comfortable to the patient than with conventional fundus photography. A time limit has been incorporated into the operative software of the HRT II that limits the duration that the laser beam can be switched on in order to further guarantee the safety to both the operator and the patient. After this time period, image acquisition will be transiently interrupted and the message "Laser Safety: laser timed out" is displayed. Imaging can continue after a set waiting period. However, this safety feature is not generally activated during normal clinical use of the instrument.

BASICS OF OPERATION

The advances incorporated in the HRT II have made clinical operation of the instrument considerably easier for the imaging technician. Each two-dimensional optical section takes about 0.025 second, and a single scan of 2 mm in depth can be performed in about 1 second. A typical imaging session with the HRT II including the pre-scan and three confocal scans can usually be obtained in under 7 seconds. The unit automatically repeats scans interrupted by blinks or large saccades so that three high-quality scans are obtained for each imaging session. The individual scans are then stored on the hard drive for later processing.

Once the three scans are stored, post-scan image processing may be carried out at any time. The software automatically aligns and averages the images to obtain a matrix of mean height measurements. The result produces the reflectance image and the topography image. After image processing is complete, the software displays both of these images with the reflectance image on the right and the topographic image on the left.

THE REFLECTANCE IMAGE

The reflectance image is a false-color image that appears similar to a photograph of the optic disc (Figure 1.3). If taken properly, the image should be clear and evenly illuminated, with sharp borders at the visible margins of the optic disc and retinal vessels. This image is the result of the summations of the two-dimensional reflectance images and is presented as a 384 X 384 pixel map illustrating the degree of reflectance from regions in the optic disc and peripapillary retina. Darker areas are regions of decreased overall reflectance, whereas lighter areas, such as the base of the cup, are areas of the greatest reflectance. This does not equate to height measurement and is purely related to the overall regional reflectance in the image. The reflectance image can be valuable in locating and drawing the contour line around the disc margin.

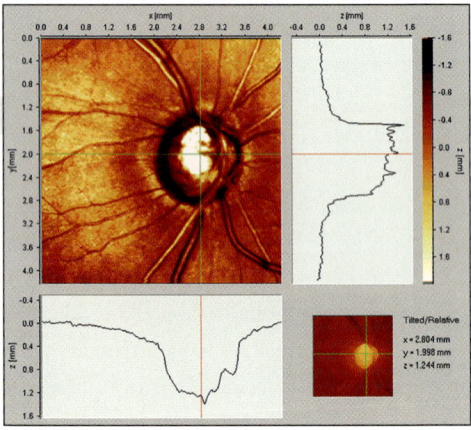

Figure 1.3

The reflectance image of the right eye of a patient with glaucoma. This false-color image has a similar appearance to an optic nerve photograph. Areas of highest reflectance, such as the base of the cup, appear brighter. In this view, the topographic image is displayed in the lower right and the cross-sectional height of the retinal surface in relation to the reflectance and topographic images are shown in the two graphs below (along the y-axis) and to the right (along the x-axis) of the reflectance image.

THE TOPOGRAPHIC IMAGE

The topographic image, in contrast to the reflectance image, relays information concerning the height of the surface contour of the optic disc and retina. This image is also false-color coded, but it is based upon the height measurement matrix constructed from the determination of the depth of maximal reflectance in the z-axis at each pixel (Figure 1.4). Pixels that appear bright in the topographic image are deeper, and dark pixels are elevated. Thus, the neuroretinal rim should appear darker than the surrounding retina and the base of the cup usually appears lightest. The topography of the optic disc may also be viewed in the 3-D view as a rotatable, three-dimensional model of the surface of the optic disc and the adjacent retina (Figure 1.5).

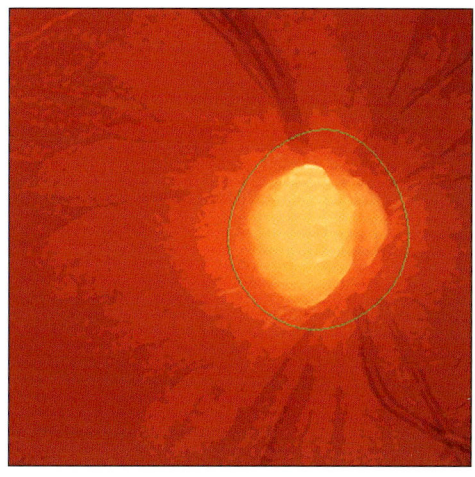

Figure 1.4

The topographic image of the same eye. This false-color image displays a 384 X 384 pixel map of the surface height. Lighter areas such as the base of the cup are deeper, while darker areas such as the surface along the retinal vessels appear darker. The contour line has been drawn around the disc margin in this image.

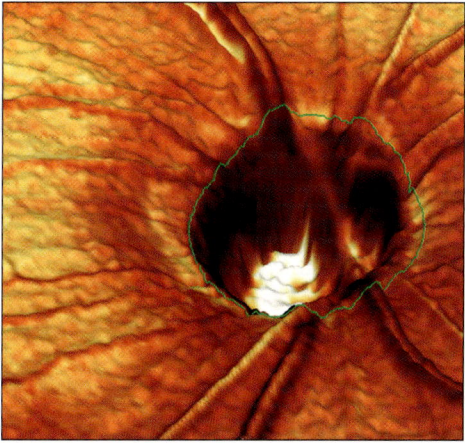

Figure 1.5

Pseudo-three-dimensional image of the optic disc. This view provides an alternative method to display contour information contained in the topographic plot. The surface characteristics of the retina and optic disc can be visualized in three dimensions by this display, which can be manually rotated.

THE REFERENCE PLANE

After the contour line is drawn around the border of the optic disc as described in Chapter 2, the HRT II software automatically places a reference plane parallel to the peripapillary retinal surface located 50 μm below the retinal surface as measured along the contour line in the papillomacular bundle (350° to 356°). The reference plane is the approximated location of the lower extent of the nerve fiber layer since the papillomacular bundle is assumed to show less change as glaucoma develops and progresses. The reference plane is used to calculate the thickness and cross-sectional area of the retinal nerve fiber layer along the contour line by subtracting retinal height as measured in the topographic image from the height of the reference plane. The height of the retina and location of the reference plane along the contour line can be viewed in the HRT II printout as a plot of the z-axis (mm) by the angle of location around the optic disc, beginning at the temporal horizontal midline of the disc and coursing clockwise in the right eye and counterclockwise in the left eye (Figure 1.6).

In addition, the parameters of area and volume of the neuroretinal rim and optic cup are also calculated based on the location of the reference plane. For both volumetric and planimetric calculations, the cup is considered to be the area of the image within the contour line that falls below the reference plane, whereas areas within the contour line that are of greater height than the reference plane are considered the neuroretinal rim (Figure 1.7). Optic disc parameters and their interpretation are reviewed in subsequent chapters.

REFERENCES

1. Zangwill LM, Weinreb RN, Berry CC, et al. The confocal scanning laser ophthalmoscopy ancillary study to the ocular hypertension treatment study: study design and baseline factors. *Am J Ophthalmol.* 2004;137:219-227.

2. Zangwill LM, Weinreb RN, Berry CC, et al. Racial differences in optic disc topography: baseline results from the confocal scanning laser ophthalmoscopy ancillary study to the ocular hypertension treatment study. *Arch Ophthalmol.* 2004;122:22-28.

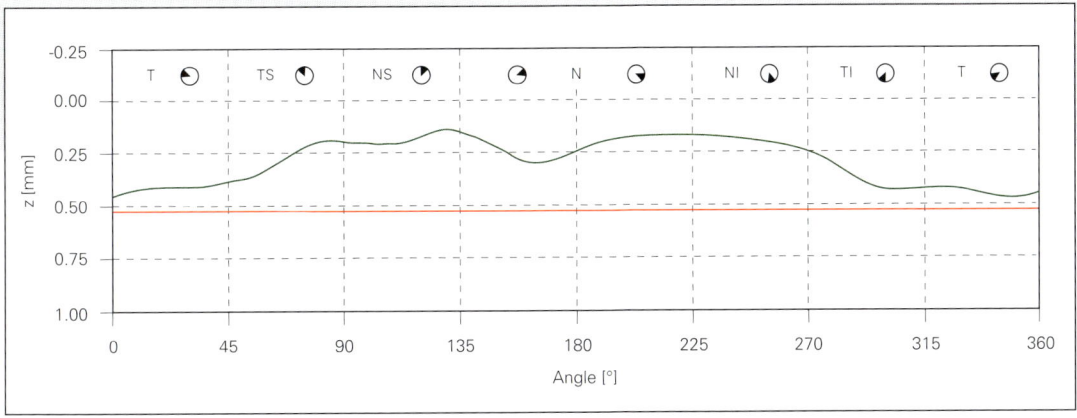

Figure 1.6

Plot of surface height around the contour line of the optic disc beginning in the temporal midline and coursing superiorly clockwise in the same eye. The green line illustrates retinal height and the red line represents the location of the reference plane place 50 μm deep to the retinal surface in the temporal peripapillary region. The thickness of the nerve fiber layer is assumed to be the differences between these two lines.

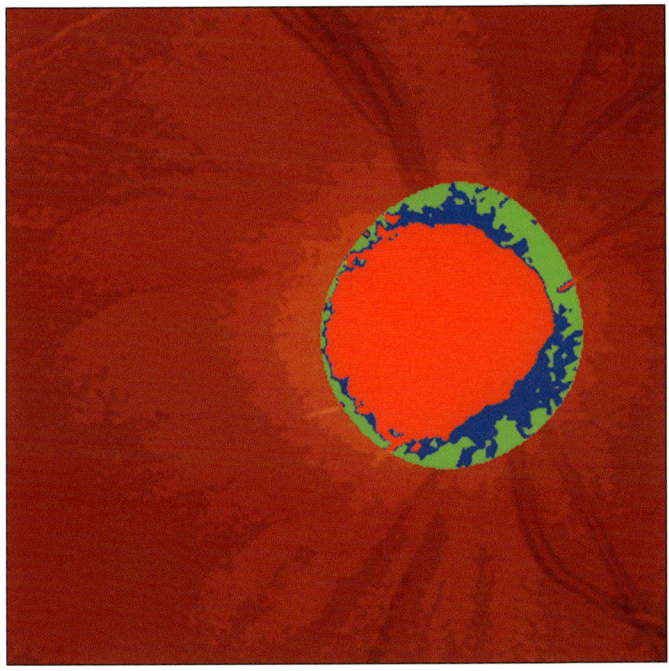

Figure 1.7

False-color coding of the area of the neuroretinal rim (blue and green) and the optic cup (red) overlaid on the topographic plot for the right eye of the same patient.

2 Using the Heidelberg Retina Tomograph II (HRT II): Image Acquisition and Accessing the Data

Murray Fingeret, OD

PRACTICAL ASPECTS OF IMAGE ACQUISITION

Patient factors

Obtaining a sharp, high-quality image with the HRT II is dependent upon several variables, including pupil size, media clarity, patient fixation, and focus. Each of these aspects of image acquisition should be assessed prior to examination and addressed when possible.

Proper patient positioning is imperative. When taking an image, the patient should be comfortably seated and the chair adjusted to the correct height to permit the forehead to fall forward naturally onto the middle of the headrest. The patient should be instructed to keep his/her forehead against the headrest at all times and look into the lens of the camera as it is brought close to the eye. The lens should be near but not touch the eyelashes, approximately 10 mm (Figure 2.1). The pupil may not need to be dilated if it is 3 to 4 mm in diameter, and the majority of patients can be imaged without dilation. Older individuals and those with cataracts are more likely to need a larger pupil size to obtain a consistent image. Younger patients with active accommodation may also be easier to image following mydriasis, as they can experience differences in accommodative status between the three image series that are automatically acquired. A poor-quality tear film will also reduce image quality. In this latter situation, the image quality degrades as the eyes remain open (Figures 2.2A, B). The first image is usually adequate, but succeeding images diminish in quality and frequently show a series of ring-type artifacts. Placing a drop of an artificial tear onto the cornea just before the image is taken often markedly improves the image quality.

ACQUIRING THE IMAGE

The first step during image acquisition with the HRT II is to enter the patient's name into the computer and to select "acquisition." The camera will enter the live mode automatically. The patient should be instructed to look straight ahead into the camera until a red box in the center of the field of view is visualized. For the right eye, the patient should look to the left of the box (toward the nose) and for the left eye, to the right (toward the nose) until a green flashing light is seen which serves as the fixation point. With proper fixation the optic nerve should appear centered in the monitor. The approximate power of the eye's refraction is dialed

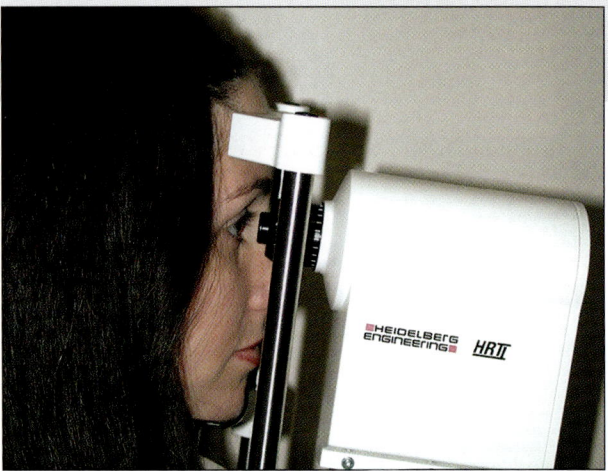

Figure 2.1

This patient is being imaged with the HRT II. Note the position of the camera to the eye and eyelashes. The camera should be near but not touch the eyelashes and be centered within the pupil.

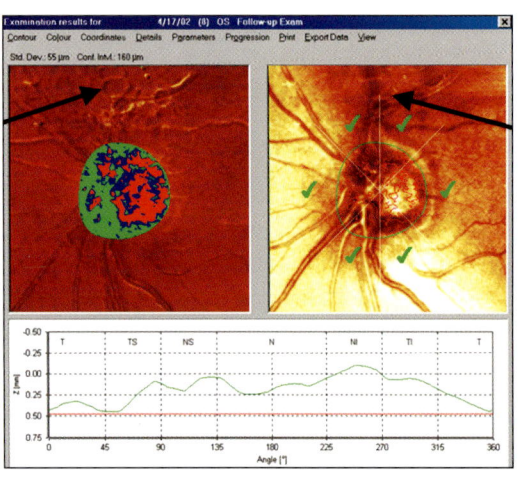

Figure 2.2A

A blurred image due to the tear film evaporating.

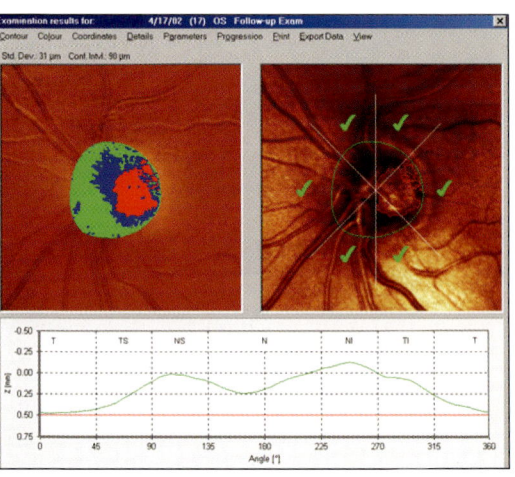

Figure 2.2B

The same patient immediately after a tear has been placed into the eye.

12 FINGERET | Using the HRT II

into the lens of the camera as the technician views the image on the monitor. The adjustable lens on the camera is moved one click at a time, with the image brightening as the retinal surface is brought into focus. A bracketing technique is used to obtain the correct focus with an extra click in either direction darkening the image and reducing the sensitivity (Figures 2.3A, B). On the monitor a live sensitivity check assists the operator. The sensitivity number decreases with improved focus with the number of blue bars increasing. The farther the blue bars extend to the right, and the lower the sensitivity number is, the better the image quality. The camera head is moved horizontally and vertically in small steps using the control dials until the image is evenly illuminated. This also enhances the image quality and improves the sensitivity values. Just before taking an image, the patient should be instructed to blink and then to hold his/her eyes open as they look at the green fixation light. When the camera switch is depressed, the camera performs an automatic pre-scan using a 4- to 6-mm depth. From the image obtained in the pre-scan, the software automatically sets the correct location of the focal plane (fine focus), the required scan depth (depth), and the proper sensitivity to obtain images with correct brightness (sensitivity). The HRT II automatically acquires three three-dimensional images with the predetermined acquisition settings. The size of the field of view is fixed at 15° x 15°, and digitization is performed in frames of 384 x 384 pixels. This ensures that with the size of the field of view for the HRT II image being 15°, the spatial resolution will be the same as the original 10° HRT images (10 µm/pixel). A comparison of HRT images with HRT II images is shown in Table 2.1.

The number of image planes acquired per series depends upon the required scan depth with 16 images per mm of scan depth. The maximum number of images taken would be 64 for a 4-mm depth. The number of images taken and depth are reported in the information section, which can be retrieved from the first screen for the patient. Automatic quality control occurs during image acquisition; if one or more of the images cannot be used for any reason (e.g., loss of fixation or blink), additional images are automatically acquired until three useful image series are obtained. The three acquired images are saved on the hard drive and the mean topography image computed.

TABLE 2.1: Comparison of the HRT and the HRT II

		HRT	HRT II
Field of View	Transverse Longitudinal	10° x 10°, 15° x 15°, or 20° x 20° 0.5 to 4.0 mm	15° x 15° 1.0 to 4.0 mm
Digital Image Size	2-D image 3-D image	256 x 256 pixels 256 x 256 x 32 voxels	384 x 384 pixels 384 x 384 x 16 to 384 x 384 x 64 voxels
Acquisition Time	2-D image 3-D image	0.032 sec 1.4 sec	0.025 sec 1.0 sec typical (2-nm depth)
Focus Range		-12 to +12 diopters	-12 to +12 diopters
Optical Resolution (limited by the eye)	Transverse Longitudinal	10 μm 300 μm	10 μm 300 μm
Digital Resolution	Transverse Longitudinal	10 to 20 μm/pixel 62 to 128 μm/plane	10 μm/pixel 62 μm/plane
Laser Source		Diode laser, 675 nm	Diode laser, 670 nm

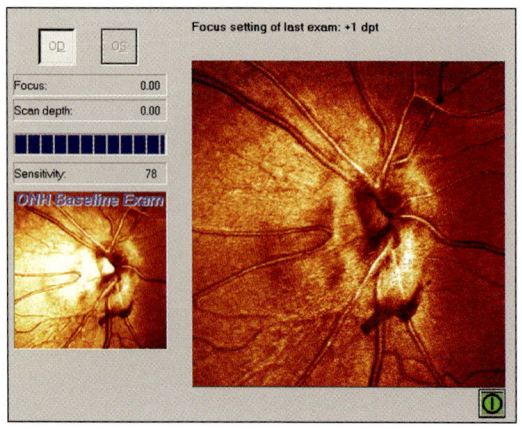

Figure 2.3A

An example of a well-focused image. The blue bars, just above the sensitivity value, are extended to the right with a sensitivity value of 78.

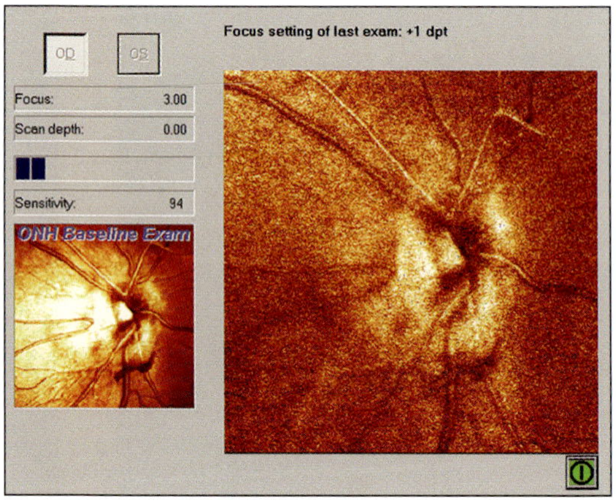

Figure 2.3B

The same eye in Figure 2.3A with the image not properly focused. The number of blue bars has decreased and the sensitivity value has increased to 94.

REVIEWING IMAGES

Once the image is taken, the digital movie can be viewed on the computer screen to assess image clarity and determine if excessive eye movements are present. Images are saved if the image appears in focus with little eye movement. It is best to ensure that the "autosave" feature is turned off so as to be able to review the image series prior to saving. Once the image is processed, the topography standard deviation appears above the contour height variation window which assesses image quality (Figure 2.4). A standard deviation (SD) under 20 μm indicates an excellent image was taken, 20 to 30 μm a very good image, and 30 to 40 μm an acceptable image. Images with a topography standard deviation above 40 μm should be interpreted with caution.

The contour line outlining the optic disc margin should be drawn next (Figures 2.5A, B, C). The contour line can be placed on either the topography or reflectance image by the placement of a series of points at the external edge of the disc border. Once three points are identified, a circle appears linking them together. Anywhere from four to six points are typically used to create the contour line, which is used for the calculation of the stereometric parameters and Moorfields analysis. Different landmarks may be used to correctly place the contour line including the appearance of the scleral ring (a change in color going from the optic disc to the retina), the bending of vessels at the disc border, and the appearance of parapapillary atrophy (Figures 2.6A, B). The nasal border of the disc may be masked due to the crowding of blood vessels, making it difficult to identify the disc edge. The interactive display aids in the proper placement of the points (Figure 2.5A). It is often helpful to draw the contour line after viewing the three-dimensional image (Figure 2.5C) or with the aid of a conventional disc photograph. The placement of the contour line occurs on both the topography and reflectance images.

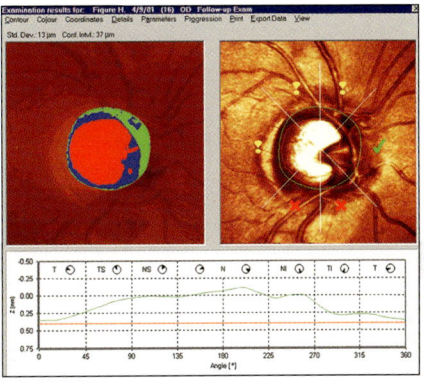

Figure 2.4

The topographic image of the same eye. This false-color image displays a 384 X 384 pixel map of the surface height. Lighter areas such as the base of the cup are deeper, while darker areas such as the surface along the retinal vessels appear darker. The contour line has been drawn around the disc margin in this image.

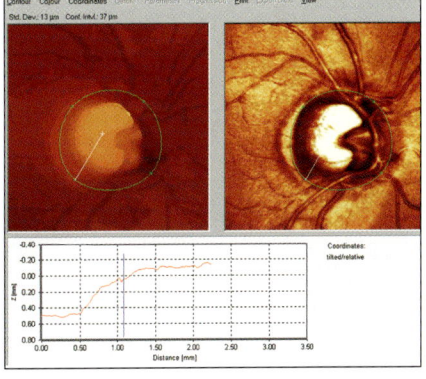

Figure 2.5A

The contour line is in the process of being drawn. Four dots have been placed at the disc margin and are connected by a circle. The topography and reflectance images are reviewed to determine whether the line is placed correctly. The dot at 8 o'clock is represented on the graph at the bottom of the screen, which shows the position of the cursor and surface height. The correct position is typically when this line plateaus off.

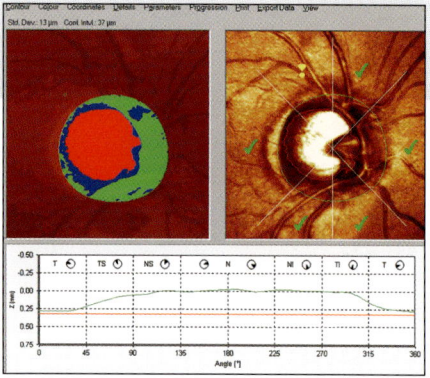

Figure 2.5B

The contour line in Figure 2.5A has been accepted and the standard deviation (SD) appears in the top left portion of the screen; the red, blue, and green appear on the topography image; and Moorfields analysis symbols are seen on the reflectance image. The mean contour height graph appears on the bottom of the screen.

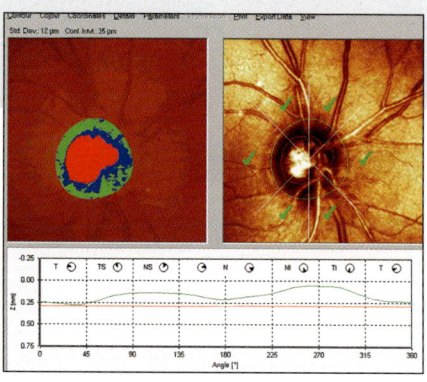

Figure 2.6A

An example of the correctly placed contour line.

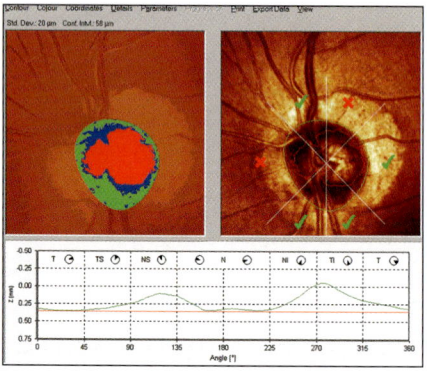

Figure 2.6B

The contour correctly placed on the edge of the disc in this optic nerve that is surrounded with parapapillary atrophy.

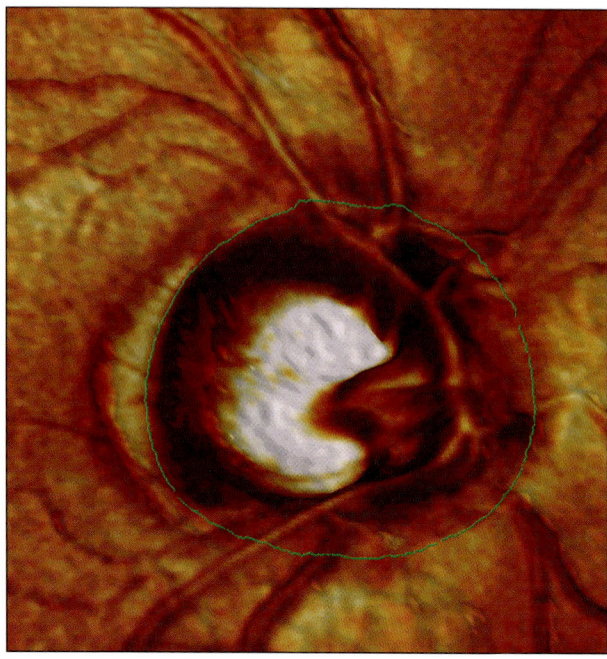

Figure 2.5C

This is the 3-D image screen of the patient in Figures 2.5A, B. The position of the contour line (green line) is best evaluated with this image.

16 FINGERET | Using the HRT II

Once the disc contour line is defined, an automatic analysis occurs with computation of the stereometric parameters, classification of the eye, and comparison to previous examinations (if prior images exist within the database). The reflectance image, on the right side of the screen, is overlaid with Moorfields analysis (Figures 2.6A, B). The reflectance image is a false-color image and appears similar to a photograph, with brighter colors representing a greater amount of reflected light. The topography image is also a false-color image and is similar to a gray scale of a visual field printout. Elevated areas typically appear darker and the lighter colors represent depressed regions. Additional colors are drawn on the topography image with red indicating the cup (area below the reference plane) and green or blue indicating neuroretinal rim tissue (area above the reference plane). Blue areas indicate the sloping rim and green areas represent nonsloping rim tissue. White areas on the topography graph indicate portions of the stable neuroretinal rim that are below the reference plane, and may be due to an incorrectly drawn contour line or severe glaucomatous injury.

The retinal surface height variation graph appears once the contour line is accepted, with the reflectance and topography image just above it on the computer screen (Figures 2.6A, B). The height variation contour line (green line) shows the height along the contour line, placed at the edge of the optic disc. It graphically displays the height of the retinal tissue along the contour line and provides a calculation of the thickness of the nerve fiber layer. On the retinal surface height contour graph, the reference line is in red with the height contour line in green. The green contour line should never go below the red reference plane (Figures 2.7A, B). If it does, then the contour line is likely not in proper position.

In the normal retina, the nerve fiber layer is thickest supero-temporally and infero-temporally so that the contour line appears as a series of hills and valleys. As the nerve fiber layer is lost in glaucoma, the retinal contour flattens and draws closer to the red reference plane. The normal retina has a classic "double hump" appearance due to the thicker nerve fiber layer at the

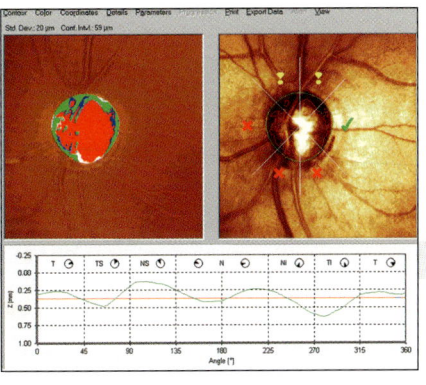

Figure 2.7A

A large optic disc is seen with a contour line not in the correct place. In the superior nasal quadrant, the contour line is just inside the edge of the disc. This is seen on the height contour map as the contour line dips below the reference plane.

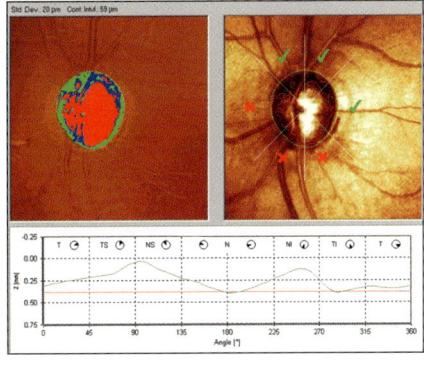

Figure 2.7B

The same optic disc as in Figure 2.7A, with the contour line modified and now in the correct position.

superior and inferior poles, but many individuals will exhibit other variations (Figures 2.8A, B). For example, the retina can be elevated along most of the contour graph, falling only in the temporal region (Figure 2.8B). The mean height contour line, drawn clockwise for the right eye and counterclockwise for the left eye, starts at the temporal region and moves superior, nasal, and inferior to finish back at the temporal location. The contour may be diminished locally (focal damage) or diffusely with an area of the contour line or the entire line falling close to the reference plane (Figures 2.9A, B, C).

Other analysis tools available on the computer screen include the three-dimensional (3-D) image (Figures 2.10A, B), interactive analysis (Figures 2.11A, B), the digital movie (Figure 2.12), stereometric parameters (Figure 2.13; Figures 2.14A, B), and Moorfields analysis (see Chapter 3). The movie plays back the image series in a rapid sequence, and appears similar to live ophthalmoscopy with the ability to stop the image at any depth (Figure 2.12). Increasing depth or a focal notch may appear as the focal plane moves deeper into the cup. The 3-D image recreates the appearance of the optic nerve and retina based upon the topographic information. The steepness of the walls of the cup or its depth is readily apparent, as is any peripapillary atrophy. The interactive display allows the horizontal and vertical profiles of the disc to be analyzed with respect to the slope, walls, and depth of the cup.

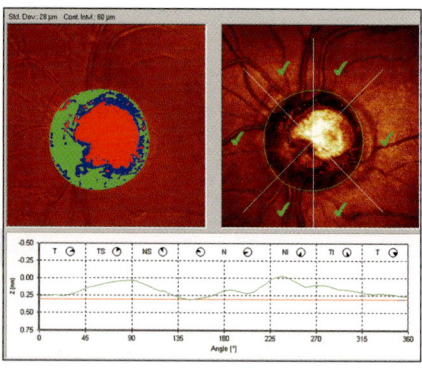

Figure 2.8A

This is an example of a large optic nerve with large physiologic cupping and a classic double-hump appearance on the contour height map.

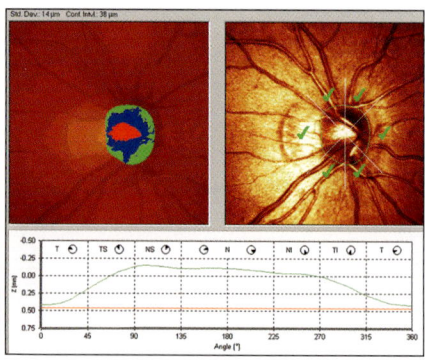

Figure 2.8B

A contour height map from a normal optic nerve in which there is only one extended hump.

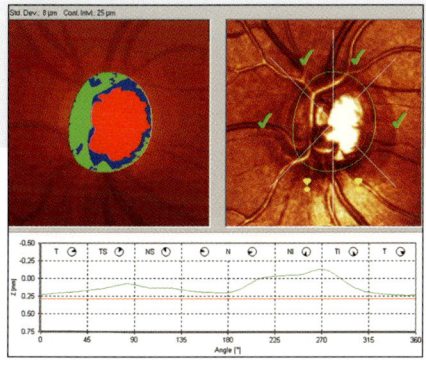

Figure 2.9A

In this individual with localized form of glaucoma, one of the humps (superior) on the contour height map is reduced.

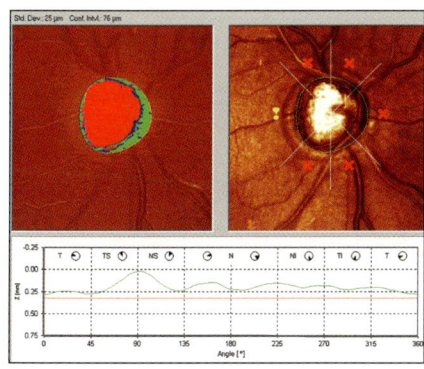

Figure 2.9B

In viewing the contour map of this individual with advanced glaucoma, both of the humps are reduced in size with the inferior one almost extinguished.

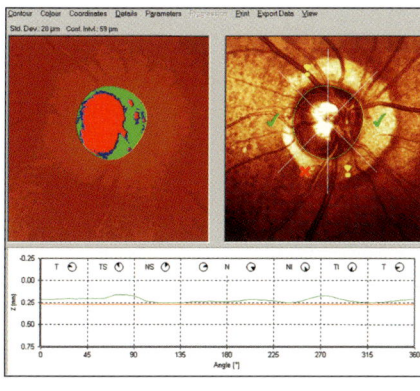

Figure 2.9C

The contour height map is almost flat in this individual with advanced glaucoma.

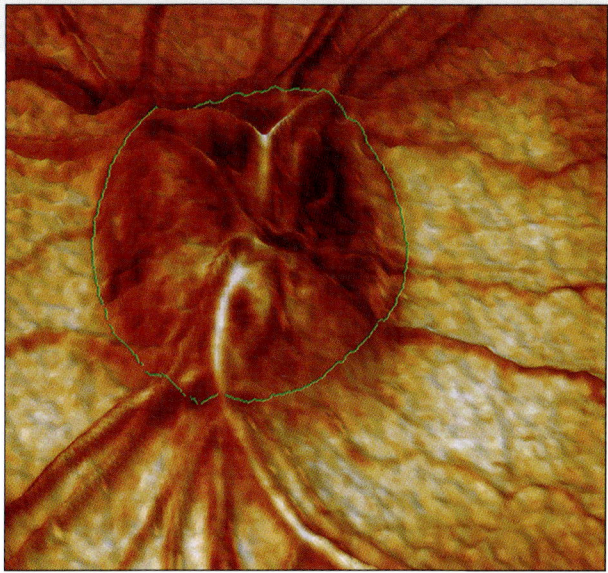

Figure 2.10A

This is a 3-D view of a person with optic nerve drusen.

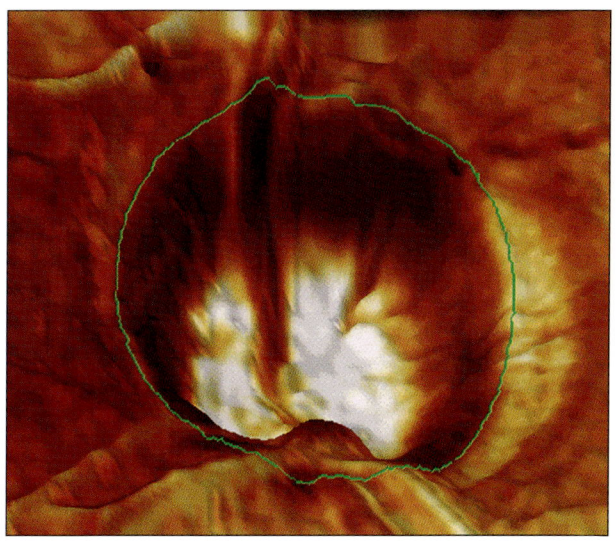

Figure 2.10B

An example of a 3-D image from a person with advanced glaucoma. Note the depth of the cup, steepness of the walls, and reduced rim tissue.

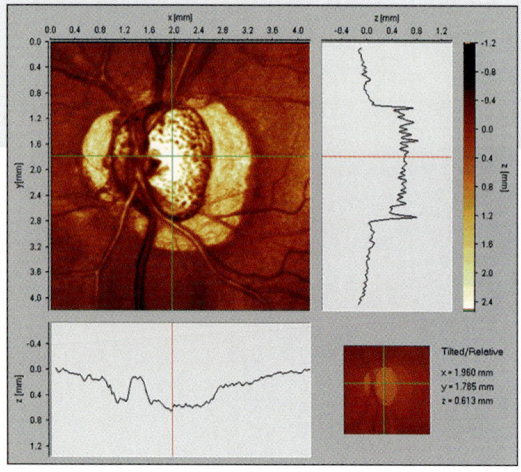 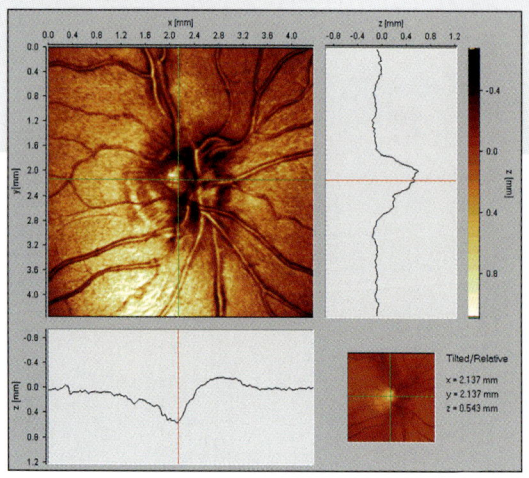

Figure 2.11A

Interactive analysis of an eye with glaucoma. Note again the depth of the cup and the vertical appearance of the walls of the cup, especially in the vertical meridian.

Figure 2.11B

Interactive analysis of a healthy optic nerve with a small cup and a subtle tilted disc. Note how the horizontal interactive line (on the bottom) raises as one moves nasally.

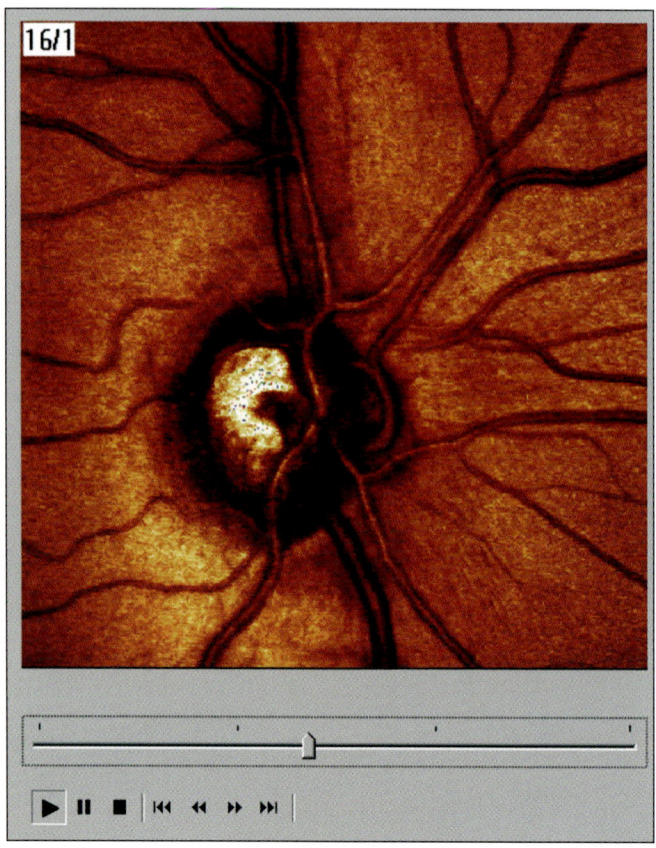

Figure 2.12

An image of the movie, in which the images are played back sequentially.

20 FINGERET | Using the HRT II

Stereometric Analysis ONH		Normal Range
Disc Area	1.858 mm²	1.69 - 2.82
Cup Area	0.906 mm²	0.26 - 1.27
Rim Area	**0.952 mm²**	**1.20 - 1.78**
Cup Volume	0.386 cmm	-0.01 - 0.49
Rim Volume	**0.161 cmm**	**0.24 - 0.49**
Cup/Disc Area Ratio	0.488	0.16 - 0.47
Linear Cup/Disc Ratio	0.698	0.36 - 0.80
Mean Cup Depth	0.424 mm	0.14 - 0.38
Maximum Cup Depth	1.235 mm	0.46 - 0.90
Cup Shape Measure	**-0.189**	**-0.27 - -0.09**
Height Variation Contour	**0.280 mm**	**0.30 - 0.47**
Mean RNFL Thickness	**0.140 mm**	**0.18 - 0.31**
RNFL Cross Sectional Area	0.680 mm²	0.95 - 1.61
Reference Height	0.307 mm	
Topography Std Dev.	15 μm	

Figure 2.13
The stereometric parameter section from the printout.

The stereometric parameters are calculated once the contour line is accepted. They quantify the size, area, and volume measurements for the optic nerve head and surrounding area. The following is a list of parameters available, either on the printout (Figure 2.13) or computer screen under parameters (Figures 2.14A, B). The definition for the stereometric parameters is given in Table 2.2.

The most important stereometric parameters are cup shape measure, rim area, rim volume, mean RNFL thickness, and height variation contour. On the printout, these parameters appear in bold print. For all the stereometric measurements, the normal range is printed next to each figure. This range represents ± 1 standard deviation from the mean. There may be individuals with glaucomatous damage whose parameters fall within the "normal range." Thus, the values are only a guide. Table 2.3 lists a normative range for the stereometric parameters. Practitioners should recognize that there is a wide overlap in many parameters between normal and affected individuals. The wide range makes classifying individual eyes based upon any one parameter difficult. Mikelberg developed a discriminant function analysis that takes into account several parameters, and classifies patients into being either normal or glaucomatous. This measure was found to have 87% sensitivity and 84% specificity. It is seen on the computer screen under the predefined segments (FSM discriminant function value). However, large optic nerves with large physiologic cups may be erroneously classified as glaucomatous. Burk also developed a discriminant function analysis, found on the computer screen under the defined segments (RB discriminant function value). Positive values are classified as normal versus outside normal limits for all other values.

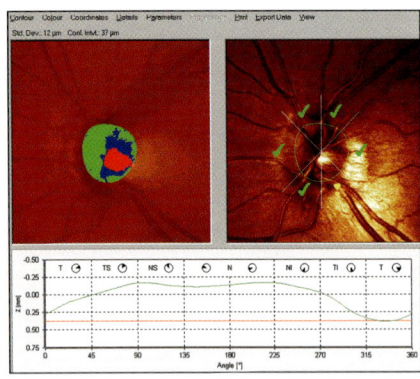

Figure 2.14A

A small optic nerve with the accompanying parameter screen shown. The optic disc size is 1.338 mm².

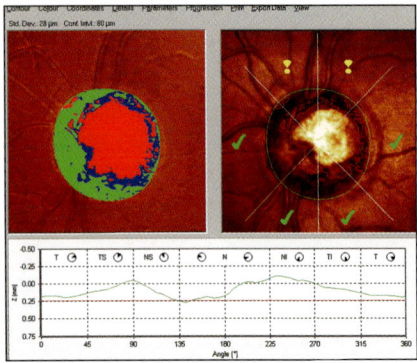

Figure 2.14B

A large optic nerve with the accompanying parameter screen shown. The disc area is 3.326 mm².

THE PRINTOUT

Analysis tools are available either on the computer screen, the printout, or both. The initial report printout (Figure 2.15A) is a summary of the different tools and contains a large amount of information. The top of the printout has patient information. The second section contains the topography image on the left side (color-coded with cup and rim information), the vertical interactive analysis in the middle, and the reflectance image overlaid with Moorfields analysis on the right. The third row has the horizontal interactive analysis on the left and the contour height line graph on the right side. On the bottom is the stereometric analysis on the left side and Moorfields analysis graph on the right. On the bottom of Moorfields classification is an overall report of how the image is classified such as Normal, Borderline, or Outside Normal Limits. The black line on the height contour graph represents the mean height of the peripapillary retinal surface. This is the zero point for the z-axis. The reference plane (red line) is displayed on the printout so that the extent of the cup is apparent. The vertical or horizontal black lines mark the edge of the disc as defined by the contour line.

Fourteen parameters are available on the printout for analysis. The most significant are in bold print. Adjacent to each parameter is the ± 1 standard deviation from the mean of the normative database. By comparing the measured parameter to the normal range, the practitioner will have an idea of where each falls within this range, based upon an appropriately positioned contour line. Seven additional parameters are available on the computer screens that are not on the printout. While the printout provides the body of information, the computer screen has supplemental information and is invaluable in assessing the HRT II image. Both should be used during image analysis. Chapter 4 will review how to use the components to interpret the image.

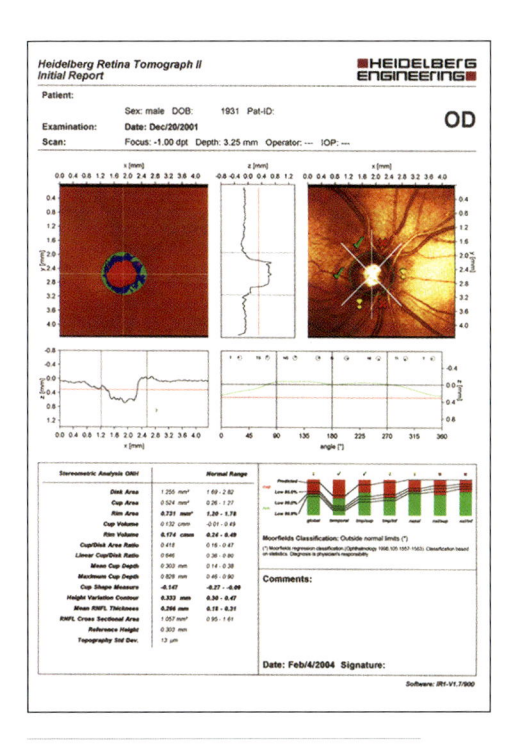

Figure 2.15A

The HRT II Initial Report. In the stereometric analysis section, the most significant parameters are in bold print.

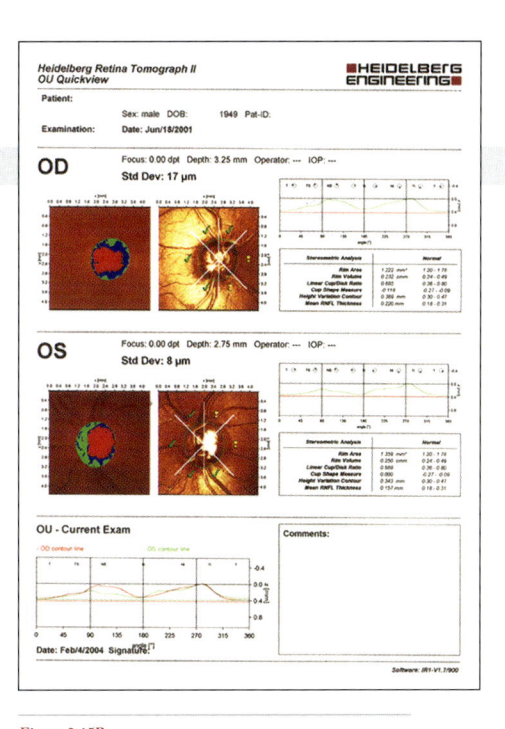

Figure 2.15B

The HRT II Quickview Report. Information for both eyes are contained on this printout, which allows a comparison between the two eyes.

Using the HRT II | FINGERET 23

OU QUICKVIEW

Another option is to use the OU Quickview printout (Figures 2.15B, C), which allows both eyes to be printed on one form, condensing the most significant information onto a single page. Differences between eyes are easily visualized with this printout. Topography and reflectance images are seen along with the standard deviation, mean contour height diagram, and the five most important parameters along with linear cup/disc ratio. On the bottom of the page are the contour lines for the two eyes, superimposed on the same scale.

One other available printout is the Follow-Up Report (Figure 2.15D). This printout is similar to the initial report, with information available as to the date of this report as well as the baseline exam, and length of time in months between reports. The other sections are similar to the initial report, with subtle differences. On the topography image, areas that have gotten worse appear in red, and areas that have improved appear in green. On the height contour line graph, the initial and baseline examinations are superimposed for comparison: the baseline in gray and the current examination in green. Stability or change can then be observed by comparing the height and shape of the lines on the graph. In the stereometric analysis section, each parameter change from the baseline is computed. Caution must be used in analyzing this section as change may occur associated with normal variability and may not be indicative of progression. Chapter 6 will go into depth in how to use the HRT in analyzing for change. The OU Quickview Report will also show change between exams as well as compute differences between the parameters. Change from baseline will be highlighted on the topography image, red for areas getting worse and green for areas showing improvement.

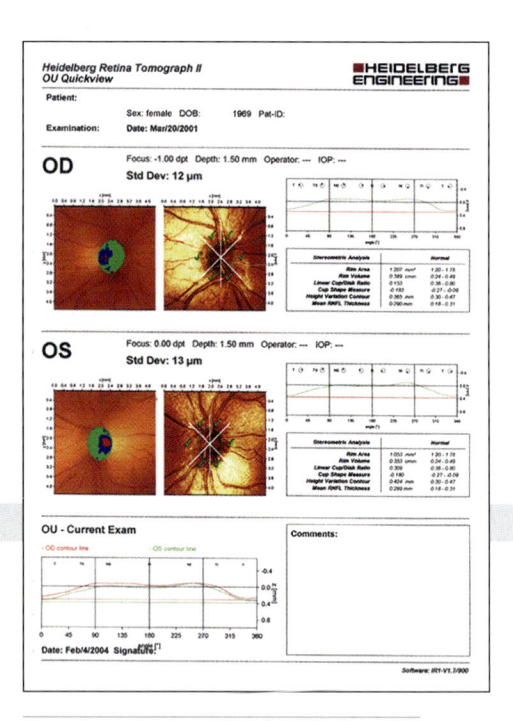

Figure 2.15C

The HRT II Quickview Report is seen for a healthy, small optic nerve.

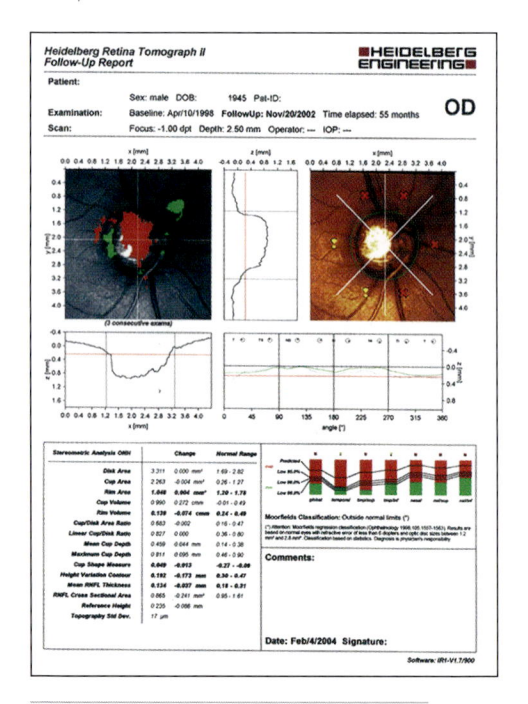

Figure 2.15D

The HRT II Follow-Up Report is seen for this patient with glaucoma. The initial image was taken on April 10, 1998, with this image taken on November 20, 2002 (55 months follow-up). The red areas in the center of the cup on the topography image signify the cup has gotten deeper. Differences among the parameters are calculated and provided. Differences among the height contour line between the baseline and most recent visit are also shown.

NEW PRINTOUT

In fall 2005, Heidelberg Engineering will introduce a new OU printout which will become the default version with older versions still available if necessary. The new printout is shown in Figure 2.16. The format is designed to provide comprehensive analysis in an easy-to-use format in order to simplify clinical interpretation. Of particular interest on this new printout is that all parameter values are automatically adjusted for age-related changes, and also for their correlation with optic disc size. Furthermore, the comparisons to a normative database are made using ethnic-specific databases. This results in a greatly reduced normative range for each parameter, making the comparisons to the normative database more sensitive for detecting abnormalities. Parameter values that fall outside the normal range will be automatically flagged as borderline or abnormal.

The printout is divided into four sections. The top section provides information on exam type (baseline or follow-up), patient demographic information (patient name, age, gender, ethnicity, etc.), and basic image information including the image quality score, focus position, and whether astigmatic lenses were used during acquisition.

The image quality score determines the overall quality of the image; the lower the score, the higher the image quality. It is based on the standard deviation value calculated at each pixel and then averaged over the entire image. The standard deviation at each pixel is calculated based on the three individual images acquired during initial scanning, and then all standard deviation values are averaged for the final standard deviation (quality) score. If the three images that are combined to create the mean image are similar (i.e., little eye movement, etc.), then the standard deviation will be low and the image quality high. Standard deviation values of 10 and below are labeled "excellent"; values between 11-20 are "very good," 21-30 are "good," 31-40 are "acceptable," 41-50 are "poor," and values above 50 are "very poor" and should be interpreted with caution. These categorical descriptions are given on the printout next to the score and color-coded. Values in the "acceptable" or better range are color-coded green, values in the "poor" range are colored yellow to indicate borderline quality, and "very poor" scores are colored red to indicate caution. It is recommended scores above 30 be repeated to try to improve quality. For some patients it may not be possible to achieve a better-quality score due to the presence of media opacity or other physical characteristic of the eye. In these cases, the best image may be used, but should be interpreted with caution.

The rest of the printout is divided into three main sections that focus on analysis related to the optic disc cup, neuroretinal rim, and RNFL respectively. The cup section shows the topography image on the baseline exam and the change analysis map on follow-up exams. The topography image provides the size, shape, and location of the cup, shown in red. The size of the optic disc is given above the topography image and is classified as small (disc sizes less than 1.6 mm^2), average (1.6 mm^2–2.6 mm^2), or large (greater than 2.6 mm^2). This section also provides two cup-related parameters, Cup/Disc Area Ratio and Cup Shape Measure. Along with the actual parameter measurements, a symmetry measure between eyes is also given. This is the ratio expressed as a percentage of OD/OS. The actual p value for each measure, based on the comparison to the appropriate ethnic-specific database, is given under each parameter. Also, a classification symbol is given next to each parameter based on the p value. If the parameter is within the 95% normal range ($p > .05$), there is a green check to indicate it is within the normal range; if the parameter is between the fifth and 0.1 percentile of the normal distribution ($p < .05$ and greater than .001), there is a yellow exclamation point to indicate borderline, and if the p value is less than the 0.1 percentile of the normal distribution, there is a red *X* indicating outside normal limits. An outside normal limits classification means that less than 0.1% (1 out of 1,000) of all normals from the database have values this low, indicating a high probability of abnormality.

The middle section of the printout provides information on the neuroretinal rim. Results of Moorfields Regression Analysis is given along with the rim parameters: Rim Area and Rim Volume. The symmetry values between eyes are also presented. The p values and classification symbols for normality for the parameters are displayed the same as for the cup parameters.

The bottom section presents information on the RNFL. The contour height graph is presented with the 95% normative range superimposed in green. As with the parameters, this normal range is determined from an ethnic-specific database after adjusting for age-related changes and optic disc size. The lightly colored solid line gives the average value for that specific age, optic disc size, and ethnicity. The yellow area represents values between the fifth and 0.1 percentile of the normal distribution ($p < .05$ and greater than .001) indicating a borderline classification, and the red area represents values below the 0.1 percentile of the normal distribution, indicating outside normal limits. There are three parameters in this section: height variation contour, mean RNFL thickness, and inter-eye symmetry. The inter-eye symmetry is the r value of the Pearson Product Correlation coefficient obtained by correlating the right and left eyes point by point along this graph. Below this parameter are the two contour height graphs plotted together. The solid black line gives the OD profile and the dashed line gives the OS profile.

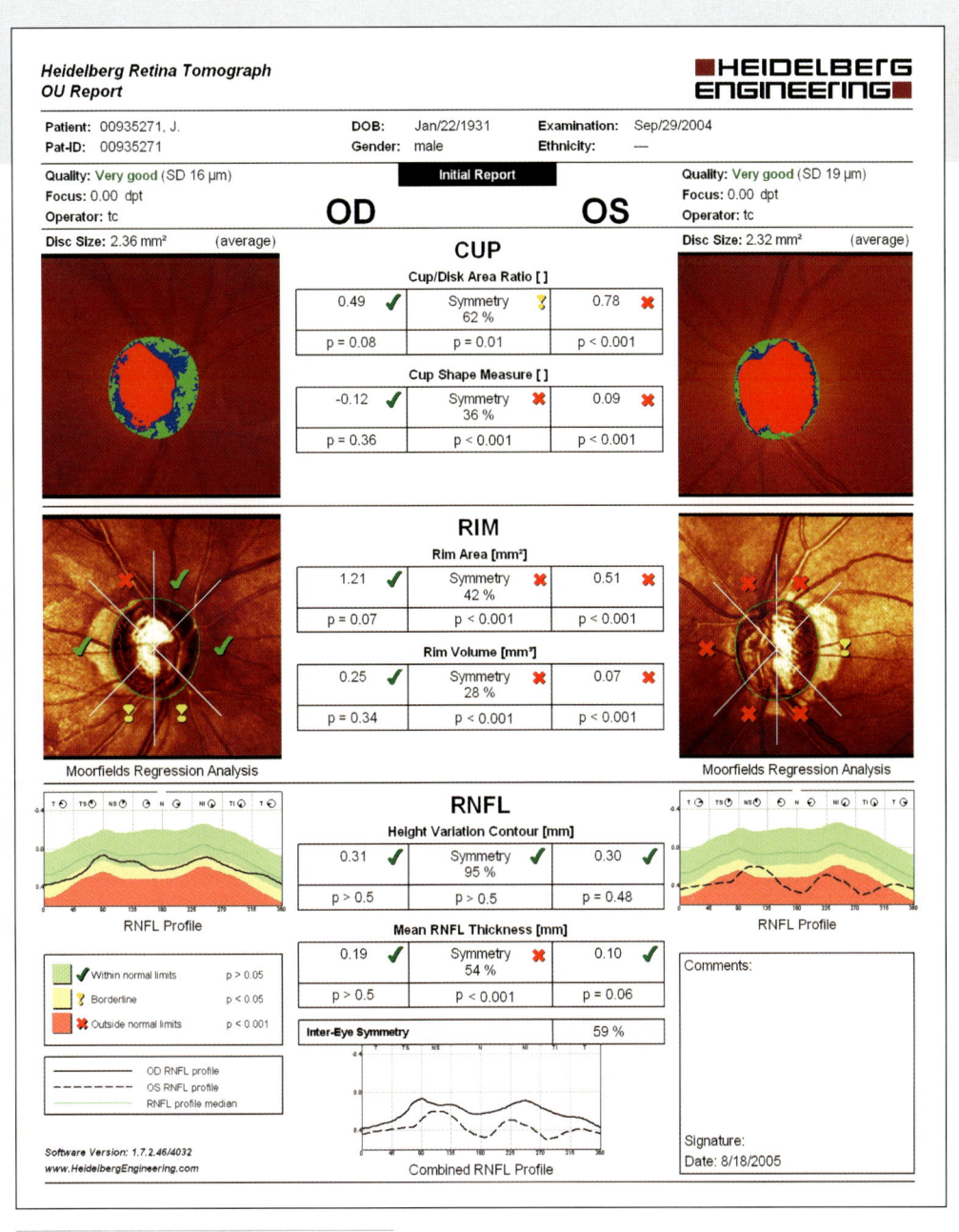

Figure 2.16
New OU printout format for the HRT software version 3.0.

TABLE 2.2: Stereometric Parameters

- **Disc Area (mm²)**
  This is the area bounded by the contour line, indicating the area of the optic disc.
- **Cup Area (mm²)**
  This is the area of optic disc cupping and is seen as the area enclosed by the contour line, which is located beneath the reference plane. It appears as a red overlay on the topography image.
- **Rim Area (mm²)**
  This is the area of the neuroretinal rim and is seen as the area enclosed by the contour line, which is located above the reference plane. It appears as either blue or green on the topography image (blue – sloping and green – stable neuroretinal rim)
- **Cup Volume (mm³)**
  The volume of optic disc cupping, defined as the volume enclosed by the contour line and located beneath the reference plane.
- **Rim Volume (mm³)**
  The volume of the neuroretinal rim, defined as the volume enclosed by the contour line and located above the reference plane.
- **Cup/Disc Area Ratio**
  Ratio of area of optic disc cupping to area of the optic disc.
- **Linear Cup/Disc Ratio**
  The average cup/disc diameter ratio calculated as the square root of the cup/disc area ratio.
- **Rim/Disc Area Ratio**
  This is the ratio between the area of neuroretinal rim and area of optic disc. This measure takes into account optic disc size.
- **Mean Cup Depth (mm)**
  This is the mean depth of the optic disc cup.
- **Maximum Cup Depth (mm)**
  This is the maximum depth of optic disc cupping.
- **Cup Shape Measure**
  This is a measure for the overall three-dimensional shape of the optic cup. It is determined as the distribution frequency of the depths inside the contour line. A normal value is on the negative side.
- **Height Variation Contour (mm)**
  This is the variation in height along the contour line, and is the difference in height between the most elevated and depressed point. This parameter decreases when nerve fiber loss occurs diffusely but increases with development of a localized nerve fiber defect.
- **Mean RNFL Thickness (mm)**
  The mean thickness of the retinal nerve fiber layer measured along the contour line, and measured relative to the reference plane.
- **RNFL Cross-Section Area (mm²)**
  This is the total cross-sectional area of the retinal nerve fiber layer along the contour line and is measured relative to the reference plane.
- **Reference Height (mm)**
  This describes the location of the reference plane, relative to the mean height of the peripapillary retinal surface.
- **Topography Standard Deviation (SD, μm)**
  This is a measure of image quality. The value, indicating a quality image, should be under 30 μm. It is the average standard deviation of all pixels in the topography image.
- **Classification**
  This description, based upon Moorfields Regression Analysis global classification, provides a guide to whether the image is suspicious. Possible classifications include "Within normal limits," "Borderline," or "Outside normal limits."
- **Maximum Contour Elevation (mm)**
  The location of the highest point of the retinal surface along the contour line, measured relative to the mean height of the peripapillary retinal surface.
- **Maximum Contour Depression (mm)**
  The location of the deepest point of the retinal surface along the contour line, measured relative to the mean height of the peripapillary retinal surface.
- **CLM Temporal - Superior (mm)**
  Contour line modulation (CLM) temporal to superior. This is the difference between the mean height of the retinal surface along the contour line in the temporal quadrant and the temporal-superior quadrant.
- **CLM Temporal - Inferior (mm)**
  Contour line modulation (CLM) temporal to inferior. This is the difference between the mean height of the retinal surface along the contour line in the temporal quadrant and the temporal-inferior quadrant.
- **Average Variability (SD, mm)**
  This is the average standard deviation of all pixels enclosed by the contour line.
- **FSM Discriminant Function Value (Mikelberg)**
  This is a discriminant value, using a formula that takes into account different parameters to classify the image as being normal or abnormal. Positive as read as "Normal" and negative "Outside normal limits."
- **RB Discriminant Function Value (Burk)**
  A different discriminant value, weighing the parameters differently from the FDM value with positive being "Normal" and negative "Outside normal limits."

TABLE 2.3: Normative Stereometric Parameters

PARAMETER	NORMAL	EARLY	MODERATE	ADVANCED
Disc Area (mm^2)	2.257 ± 0.563	2.345 ± 0.569	2.310 ± 0.554	2.261 ± 0.461
Cup Area (mm^2)	0.768 ± 0.505	0.953 ± 0.594	1.051 ± 0.647	1.445 ± 0.562
Rim Area (mm^2)	1.489 ± 0.291	1.393 ± 0.340	1.260 ± 0.415	0.817 ± 0.334
Cup Volume (mm^3)	0.240 ± 0.245	0.294 ± 0.270	0.334 ± 0.318	0.543 ± 0.425
Rim Volume (mm^3)	0.362 ± 0.124	0.323 ± 0.156	0.262 ± 0.139	0.128 ± 0.096
Cup/Disc Area Ratio	0.314 ± 0.152	0.380 ± 0.179	0.430 ± 0.203	0.621 ± 0.189
Mean Cup Depth (mm)	0.262 ± 0.118	0.279 ± 0.115	0.289 ± 0.130	0.366 ± 0.182
Maximum Cup Depth (mm)	0.679 ± 0.223	0.680 ± 0.210	0.674 ± 0.249	0.720 ± 0.276
Cup Shape Measure	-0.181 ± 0.092	-0.147 ± 0.098	-0.122 ± 0.095	-0.036 ± 0.096
Height Variation Contour (mm)	0.384 ± 0.087	0.364 ± 0.100	0.330 ± 0.108	0.256 ± 0.090
Mean RNFL Thickness (mm)	0.384 ± 0.063	0.217 ± 0.076	0.182 ± 0.086	0.130 ± 0.061
RNFL Cross-Sectional Area (mm^2)	1.282 ± 0.328	1.155 ± 0.396	0.957 ± 0.440	0.679 ± 0.302

Burk R. [Laser Scanning Tomography: Interpretation of the HRTII printout.] Laser Scanning Tomographie: Interpretation der Ausdrucke des Heidelberg Retina Tomographen HRTII. *Z prakt Augenheilkd* 2001;22:183-190.

REFERENCES

1. Mikelberg FS, Parfitt CM, Swindale NV, Graham SL, Drance SM, Gosine R. Ability of the Heidelberg Retina Tomograph to detect early glaucomatous visual field loss. *J Glaucoma*. 1995;4:242-247.

2. Burk R. Laser Scanning Tomographé: Interpretation der Ausdrucke des Heidelberg Retina Tomographen HRT II. *Z prakt Augenheilkd* [Laser scanning tomography: interpretation of the HRT II printout]. 2001;22:183-190.

3. Iester M, Broadway DC, Mikelberg FS, Drance SM. A comparison of healthy, ocular hypertensive, and glaucomatous optic disc topographic parameters. *J Glaucoma*. 1997;6:363-370.

4. Iester M, Mikelberg FS, Drance SM. The effect of optic disc size on diagnostic precision with the Heidelberg Retina Tomograph. *Ophthalmology*. 1997;104:545-548.

5. Bathija R, Zangwill L, Berry CC, Sample PA, Weinreb RN. Detection of early glaucomatous structural damage with confocal scanning laser tomography. *J Glaucoma*. 1998;7:121-127.

TABLE 2.4: Features Available on Computer or Printout

ANALYSIS TOOL	COMPUTER SCREEN	PRINTOUT	BOTH
Topography Image			XX
Reflective Image			XX
Interactive Analysis			XX
Height Contour Graph			XX
Moorfields Analysis	Numeric data on computer only		XX
Stereometric Parameters	Increased parameters with computer		XX
3-D Analysis	XX		
Movie	XX		
Progression Analysis	XX Glaucoma Change Probability		XX

3 Moorfields Regression Analysis

David F. Garway-Heath, MD, FRCOphth

INTRODUCTION

It is well established that structural changes at the optic nerve head (ONH) are an early and prominent feature of the glaucomatous disease process, so it is to be expected that measurements of ONH structure should be able to distinguish between glaucomatous and healthy nerves. The HRT II derives a large number of measurement parameters, both for the ONH as a whole ("global") and for more localized ONH regions ("predefined segments") (see Chapter 2). Different mathematical approaches have been applied to the problem of deriving a suitable algorithm that can make best use of all the measurement data to distinguish between normal and glaucomatous eyes. The most frequent approach is to take a group of healthy nonglaucomatous eyes and a group of glaucomatous eyes and submit all the measurements generated by the HRT to a linear discriminant analysis.[1,2] The output of such an analysis is a linear combination of the parameters that best distinguish between the two groups. This approach makes no assumptions about the parameters that are most likely to be useful, but the algorithm derived by the analysis is sensitive to the composition of the two subject groups taken as representative of "normal" and "glaucomatous."

An alternative approach is that taken with Moorfields Regression Analysis (MRA). The form of the analysis was derived from a prior knowledge of physiological relationships, i.e., the dependence of neuroretinal rim area on optic disc size,[3,4] the possibility that neuroretinal rim area may decline with age,[5,6] and knowledge of the glaucomatous process (e.g., narrowing of the neuroretinal rim).[7,8] Although narrowing of the rim is said to occur preferentially in some regions of the ONH, it may occur in any region. For this reason, the algorithm was based on an analysis of all segments of the ONH. The approach was first applied to planimetry (measurements from ONH photographs)[9] and then to HRT images.[10]

The algorithm used in the MRA is derived from measurement data taken from a group of 112 normal eyes. Any ONH that is determined to be "outside normal limits" is not necessarily glaucomatous but is statistically outside the normal ranges for the group of eyes in the normative database. The decision as to whether "outside normal limits" represents "glaucoma" is a clinical judgment made by considering all clinical information together.

SETTING NORMAL LIMITS

It is well established that neuroretinal rim area is related physiologically to ONH size.[3,4] This relationship is illustrated in Figure 3.1 for the eyes in the HRT II database. There is a tendency for the variability in neuroretinal rim area measurements to increase as the measurements themselves increase.

A logarithmic transformation is made to normalize the variability distribution. MRA makes use of the relationship between log neuroretinal rim area and optic disc area to define the normal ranges. Figure 3.2 illustrates the linear regression line between log neuroretinal rim area and optic disc area (marked "50%"). This is the "average" or "predicted" relationship between log neuroretinal rim area and optic disc area. The lower three lines represent the lower 95.0%, 99.0%, and 99.9% prediction intervals for the same relationship. Thus, for the 95.0% prediction interval, 95.0% of normal eyes would be expected to have a neuroretinal rim area above that interval line. The same reasoning applies to the 99.0% and 99.9% prediction intervals. These intervals are calculated for the ONH as a whole and for each of the six predefined sectors.

The classification for each ONH segment is displayed on the reflectivity image. A red X denotes "outside normal limits," a yellow exclamation mark denotes "borderline," and a green check denotes "within normal limits" (Figure 3.3).

The prediction intervals for neuroretinal rim area should be regarded in the same way as the probability symbols for abnormality in the reports from automated perimeters. The closer the top of the green bar gets to the lower prediction intervals, the greater the probability that the rim area is abnormal. The MRA Report given in the HRT II software enables a visual inspection of where the neuroretinal rim area lies in relation to the normal ranges (Figure 3.4).

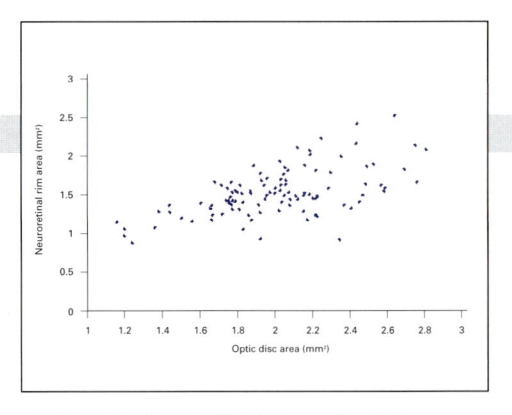

Figure 3.1

The physiological relationship between neuroretinal rim area and optic disc size in the eyes in the MRA normative database.

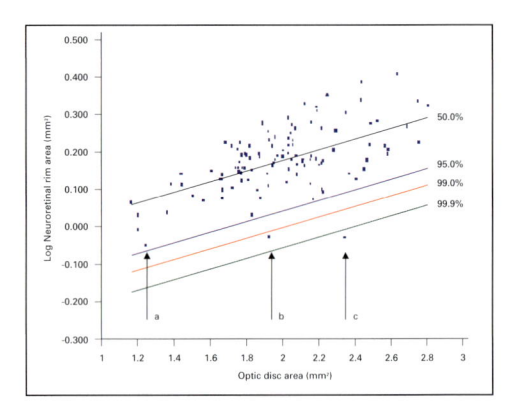

Figure 3.2

Plot of log neuroretinal rim area against optic disc area for the eyes in the MRA normative database, displaying the linear regression line and the lower 95.0%, 99.0%, and 99.9% prediction intervals. Three eyes with similar neuroretinal rim area are marked (a, b, and c). The neuroretinal rim area for "a" falls within the normal range because the optic disc is small. That for "b" falls between the 99.0% and 99.9% prediction intervals because the optic disc is of normal size. That for "c" falls below the 99.9% prediction interval because the optic disc is large. These are the lines marked on the Moorfields Regression Analysis Report given in the HRT II software, shown in Figure 3.3.

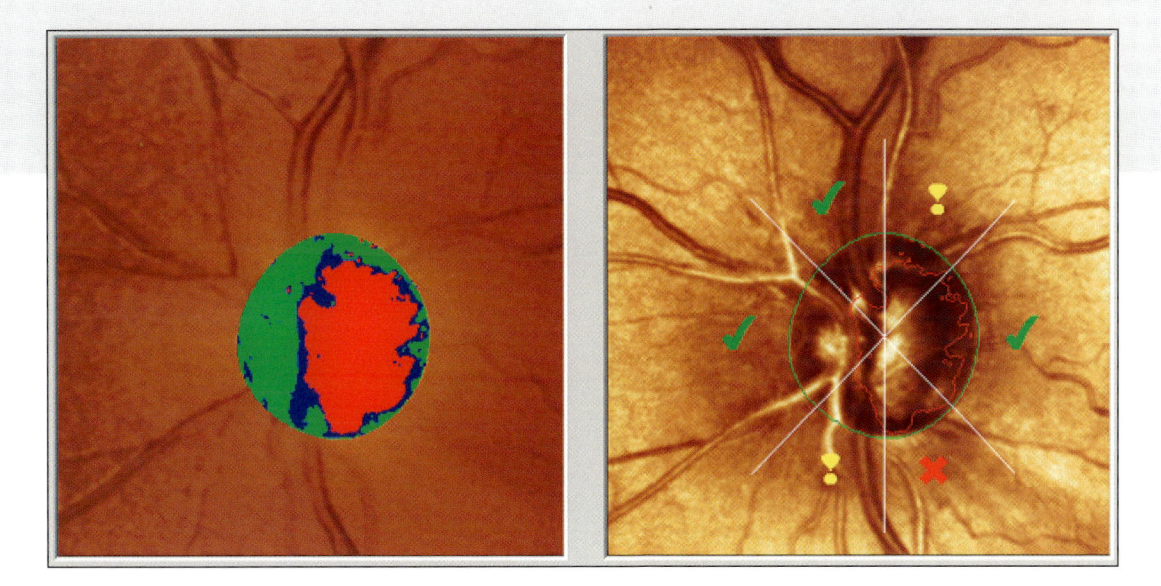

Figure 3.3

An example of a glaucomatous eye in which the neuroretinal rim area in some optic disc segments lies "within normal limits" (green check), some are "borderline" (yellow exclamation mark), and one is "outside normal limits" (red X).

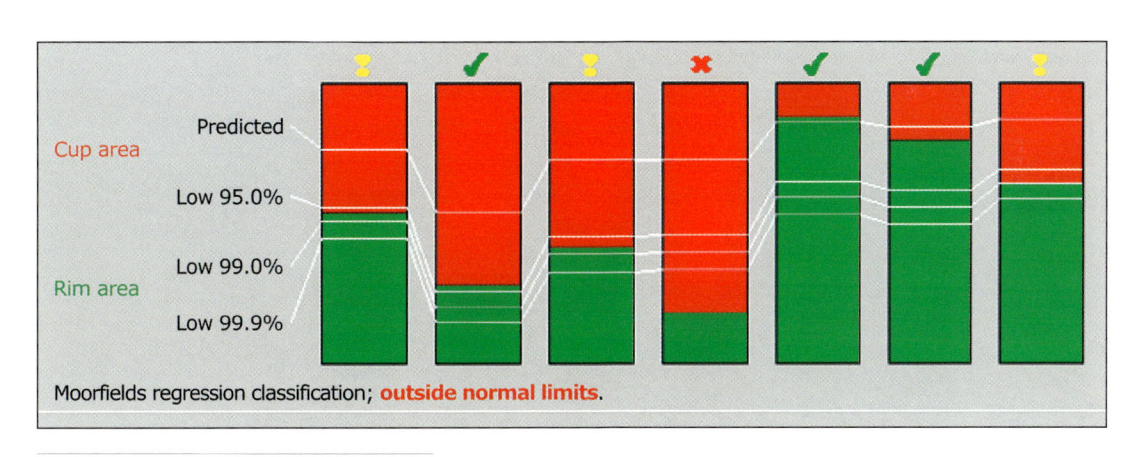

Figure 3.4

MRA: The neuroretinal rim area (in green) and optic cup area (in red) are displayed as a series of bars for the whole disc (leftmost) and each predefined segment (left to right: temporal, supero-temporal, infero-temporal, nasal, supero-nasal, and infero-nasal). The narrower the neuroretinal rim, the shorter the green bar and the nearer the top of the bar gets to the lower prediction intervals. If the top of the green bar lies above the 95.0% prediction interval, then the disc or disc segment is classified as "within normal limits." If the top of the green bar lies between the 95.0% and 99.9% prediction intervals, then the disc or disc segment is classified as "borderline." And if the top of the green bar lies below the 99.9% prediction interval, then the disc or disc segment is classified as "outside normal limits." The most abnormal of the seven classifications (whole disc and six predefined segments) gives the overall classification for the optic disc.

In the subjects in the normal database, the neuroretinal rim area was also found to be dependent on subject age for the global measurement and in the temporal and supero-temporal measurements. Figure 3.5 illustrates this relationship for the global neuroretinal rim area. Subject age is taken into account when calculating the prediction intervals for global, temporal, and supero-temporal neuroretinal rim area in the HRT II software.

INTERPRETING MOORFIELDS REGRESSION ANALYSIS

No commercially available imaging device is able to discriminate perfectly between normal and glaucomatous eyes—there is an overlap in measurements between the two. This is illustrated in Figure 3.6. At certain levels of neuroretinal rim area there is, therefore, uncertainty as to whether the measurement is within or outside normal limits. In MRA, this zone of uncertainty has been designated "borderline."

MRA has been applied to a large number of normal and glaucomatous eyes from four different research centers.[11] HRT II classification of normal and glaucomatous eyes is given in Table 3.1. Similar results have been reported in a more recent publication.[12]

Table 3.1 gives proportions of normal and glaucomatous eyes classified into each HRT II classification group. However, the actual numbers of normal and glaucomatous subjects in each classification group depend on the prevalence of glaucoma in the population undergoing examination. Figure 3.7 illustrates the case of a 2.4% glaucoma prevalence.[13]

Table 3.2 gives the proportions of eyes, by true diagnosis, in each HRT classification group for a population with a 2.4% glaucoma prevalence. Note that only 4% of borderline cases will have glaucoma. Also note that because of the much larger number of normal subjects in the general population, even a low misclassification rate of 7% results (as it would with other imaging devices) in more normal subjects being misclassified as "outside normal limits" than glaucomatous subjects being correctly classified as "outside normal limits."

Whereas a 2.4% prevalence might represent the situation encountered when screening the general population, most clinicians examine patients that have been preselected in some way. In the UK, a typical referral population has a glaucoma prevalence of at least 30%. In this setting the proportions of normal and glaucomatous eyes designated as "borderline" are more balanced. This is illustrated in Figure 3.8. The proportions of normal and glaucomatous eyes in each HRT classification group is given in Table 3.3.

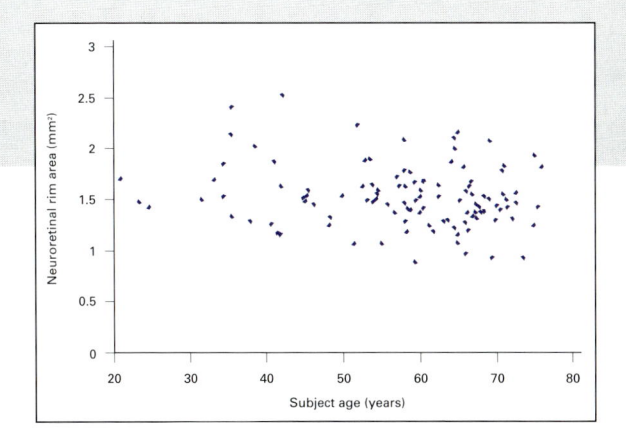

Figure 3.5

Plot of the global neuroretinal rim area against age in the eyes in the MRA normative database.

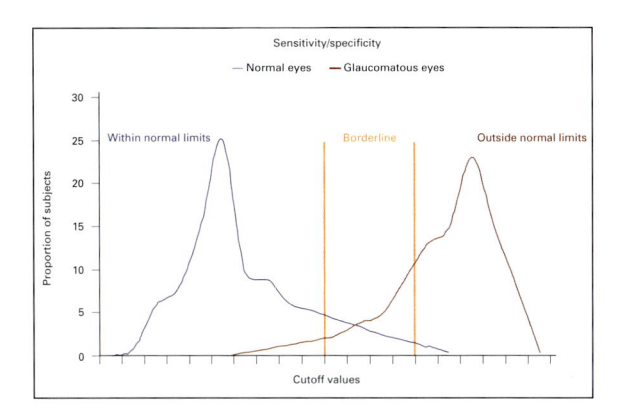

Figure 3.6

Plot of the distribution of normal and glaucomatous eyes at various cutoff levels of neuroretinal rim area. Note the overlap between the two.

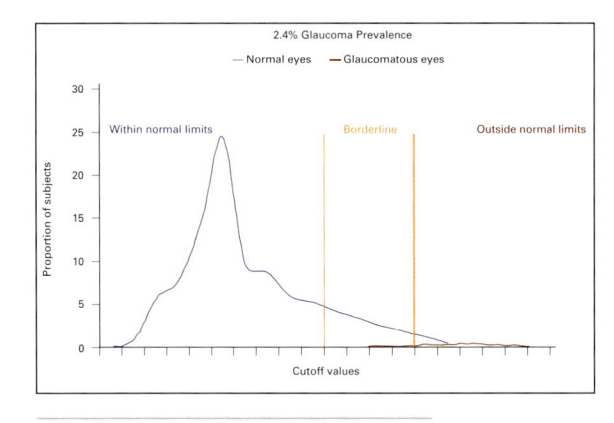

Figure 3.7

Relative proportions of normal and glaucomatous eyes in the "within normal limits," "borderline," and "outside normal limits" classification zones for a population with a glaucoma prevalence of 2.4%.

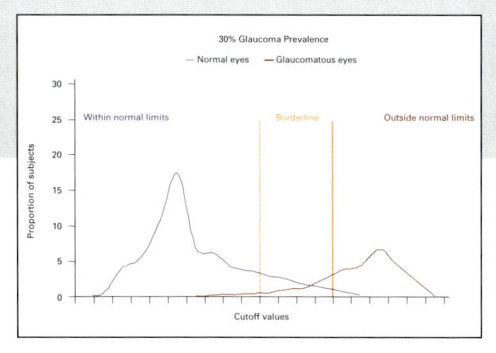

Figure 3.8

Relative proportions of normal and glaucomatous eyes in the "within normal limits," "borderline," and "outside normal limits" classification zones for a population with a glaucoma prevalence of 30%.

TABLE 3.1: HRT II classification of 321 normal and 283 eyes with early glaucoma.

	Within normal limits	Borderline	Outside normal limits
Normal	79%	14%	7%
Glaucoma	14%	19%	67%

TABLE 3.2: Proportion of eyes in each HRT classification group by true diagnosis for a glaucoma prevalence of 2.4%.

	True normal (%)	True glaucoma (%)
HRT "within normal limits"	>99	<1
HRT "borderline"	96	4
HRT "outside normal limits"	81	19

TABLE 3.3: Proportion of eyes in each HRT classification group by true diagnosis for a glaucoma prevalence of 30%.

	True normal (%)	True glaucoma (%)
HRT "within normal limits"	93	7
HRT "borderline"	63	37
HRT "outside normal limits"	20	80

It can be seen from Tables 3.1 and 3.3 that the MRA greatly aids the correct classification of individual subjects. However, as with intraocular pressure measurements and visual field testing, no single test used on its own is sufficiently precise for the diagnosis of glaucoma. Thus, measurement data from all sources available (including history and examination) need to be integrated to obtain a probability of disease status. Table 3.4 illustrates the effect of taking intraocular pressure into account when interpreting the HRT classification for a population with a 2.4% glaucoma prevalence. The calculations assume a prevalence of ocular hypertension (OHT, intraocular pressure above 21 mm Hg in a nonglaucomatous eye) of 3.7%[13] and a prevalence of normal tension glaucoma of 40% of the glaucomatous population.

Table 3.5 gives a similar analysis for a population with a 30% prevalence of glaucoma. It can be seen from these examples that MRA findings are best interpreted in the clinical context, together with all findings of history and examination.

NORMATIVE DATABASE

Any classification system that relies on normative data is sensitive to the composition of the normative database. It is therefore important to know how similar an individual patient is to the composition of the normative database when assessing classification results. If a patient deviates from the characteristics of subjects in the database, then the classification results should be interpreted cautiously. Important characteristics of the MRA normative database are that all subjects were white ("Caucasian ethnic group") and with ametropia of < 6 diopters. The range of optic disc size in the database reflects that of the population from which the normal volunteers were derived, with an upper limit of around 2.80 mm^2. There were also few tilted optic discs.

The MRA classification should be used cautiously in subjects that are nonwhite, although a recent publication has demonstrated similar specificity of MRA in black and white Americans.[14] Racial differences in normative values may necessitate ethnic-specific cutoffs to optimize disease detection strategies.

Disc size is taken into account in MRA. However, some residual effect of disc size on classification remains,[12] and the MRA classification in discs larger than 2.80 mm^2 may be less specific. Care should also be taken in assessing eyes with a high refractive error, or that have marked disc tilt. Heidelberg Engineering is currently expanding the HRT II normative database to include more normal subjects from a wide range of ethnic backgrounds and to increase the range of optic disc size. If differences in the neuroretinal rim/optic disc size relationship are found between different ethnic groups, then ethnicity-specific normative databases will be derived.

In the same way that certain features may give rise to a false-positive classification of a normal ONH (such as a large ONH), certain features of glaucomatous ONHs may give rise to false-negative classification. The most frequent of these is shallow cupping in the presence of marked parapapillary atrophy. In these cases the optic disc is often clearly abnormal on the clinical examination.

False-negative and false-positive classification may occur if the ONH margin (contour line) is incorrectly drawn. The ONH margin is defined as the inner margin of the scleral ring of Elschnig.

TABLE 3.4: The proportion of subjects with true glaucoma, with and without OHT, in each HRT classification group for a population with a 2.4% glaucoma prevalence.

	With OHT (%)	Without OHT (%)
HRT "within normal limits"	7	<1
HRT "borderline"	35	1
HRT "outside normal limits"	79	9

TABLE 3.5: The proportion of subjects with true glaucoma, with and without OHT, in each HRT classification group for a population with a 30% glaucoma prevalence.

	With OHT (%)	Without OHT (%)
HRT "within normal limits"	55	3
HRT "borderline"	90	19
HRT "outside normal limits"	99	63

OPTIC DISC / VISUAL FIELD TOPOGRAPHIC RELATIONSHIP

A particular advantage of MRA is the sectoral nature of the analysis, so that it is possible to compare the sectoral neuroretinal rim area (length of the green bar in relation to the prediction intervals) to the corresponding regions of the visual field on the basis of known anatomy.[15] Figure 3.9 illustrates the correspondence between the HRT predefined segments and the visual field.

Figure 3.10 illustrates an example of a 67-year-old subject with ocular hypertension who developed an infero-temporal notch in the optic disc with corresponding superior paracentral arcuate visual field loss.

CONCLUSION

Moorfields Regression Analysis provides clinically useful information regarding the topography of the optic disc in comparison to a normative database and aids the correct classification of individual patients. The appearance of the optic disc and the results of this analysis should be evaluated in the context of the clinical examination and tests of visual function.

REFERENCES

1. Mikelberg FS, Parfitt CM, Swindale NV, Graham SL, Drance SM, Gosine R. Ability of the Heidelberg Retina Tomograph to detect early glaucomatous visual field loss. *J Glaucoma*. 1995;4:242-247.
2. Bathija R, Zangwill L, Berry CC, Sample PA, Weinreb RN. Detection of early glaucomatous structural damage with confocal scanning laser tomography. *J Glaucoma*. 1998;7:121-127.
3. Betz P, Camps F, Collignon-Brach C, Weekers R. Stereophotography and photogrammetry of the physiological cup of the disc [in French]. *J Fr Ophtalmol*. 1981;4:193-203.
4. Jonas JB, Gusek GC, Naumann GO. Optic disc, cup and neuroretinal rim size, configuration and correlations in normal eyes [published errata appear in *Invest Ophthalmol Vis Sci* 1991;32:1893 and 1992;32:474-475]. *Invest Ophthalmol Vis Sci*. 1988;29:1151-1158.
5. Pickard R. The alteration in size of the normal optic disc cup. *Br J Ophthalmol*. 1948;32:355-361.
6. Garway-Heath DF, Wollstein G, Hitchings RA. Aging changes of the optic nerve head in relation to open angle glaucoma. *Br J Ophthalmol*. 1997;81:840-845.
7. Read RM, Spaeth GL. The practical clinical appraisal of the optic disc in glaucoma: the natural history of cup progression and some specific disc-field correlations. *Trans Am Acad Ophthalmol Otolaryngol*. 1974;78:255-267.
8. Tuulonen A, Airaksinen PJ. Initial glaucomatous optic disk and retinal nerve fiber layer abnormalities and their progression. *Am J Ophthalmol*. 1991;111:485-490.
9. Garway-Heath DF, Hitchings RA. Quantitative evaluation of the optic nerve head in early glaucoma. *Br J Ophthalmol*. 1998;82:352-361.
10. Wollstein G, Garway-Heath DF, Hitchings RA. Identification of early glaucoma cases with the scanning laser ophthalmoscope. *Ophthalmology*. 1998;105:1557-1563.
11. Ally F, Garway-Heath DF, Mardin CY, et al. Comparison of algorithms used to classify eyes by means of Heidelberg Retina Tomograph measurement data [ARVO abstract]. *Invest Ophthalmol Vis Sci*. 2001;42:S118. Abstract 635.
12. Ford BA, Artes PH, McCormick TA, Nicolela MT, LeBlanc RP, Chauhan BC. Comparison of data analysis tools for detection of glaucoma with the Heidelberg Retina Tomograph. *Ophthalmology*. 2003;110:1145-1150.
13. Mitchell P, Smith W, Attebo K, Healey PR. Prevalence of open-angle glaucoma in Australia. The Blue Mountains Eye Study. *Ophthalmology*. 1996;103:1661-1669.
14. Girkin CA, McGwin G Jr, Xie A, Deleon-Ortega J. Differences in optic disc topography between black and white normal subjects. *Ophthalmology*. 2005;112:33-39.
15. Garway-Heath DF, Poinoosawmy D, Fitzke FW, Hitchings RA. Mapping the visual field to the optic disc in normal tension glaucoma eyes. *Ophthalmology*. 2000;107:1809-1815.

Figure 3.9

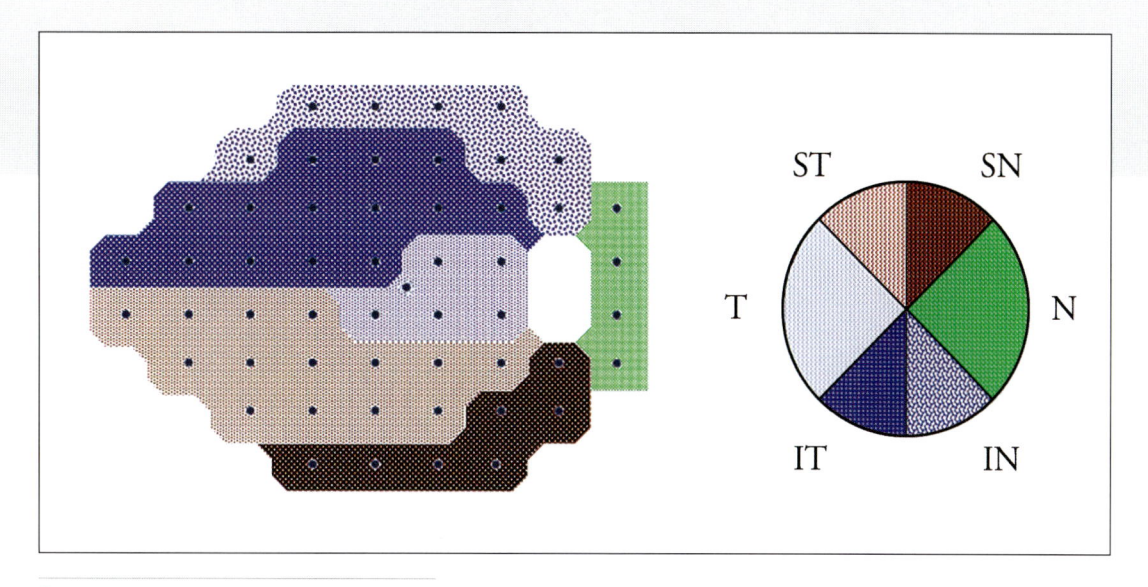

The Humphrey 24-2 visual field grid for a right eye divided into regions that correspond with the HRT II predefined ONH sectors.

(T = Temporal, ST = Supero-temporal,
IT = Infero-temporal, N = Nasal,
SN = Supero-nasal, IN = Infero-nasal)

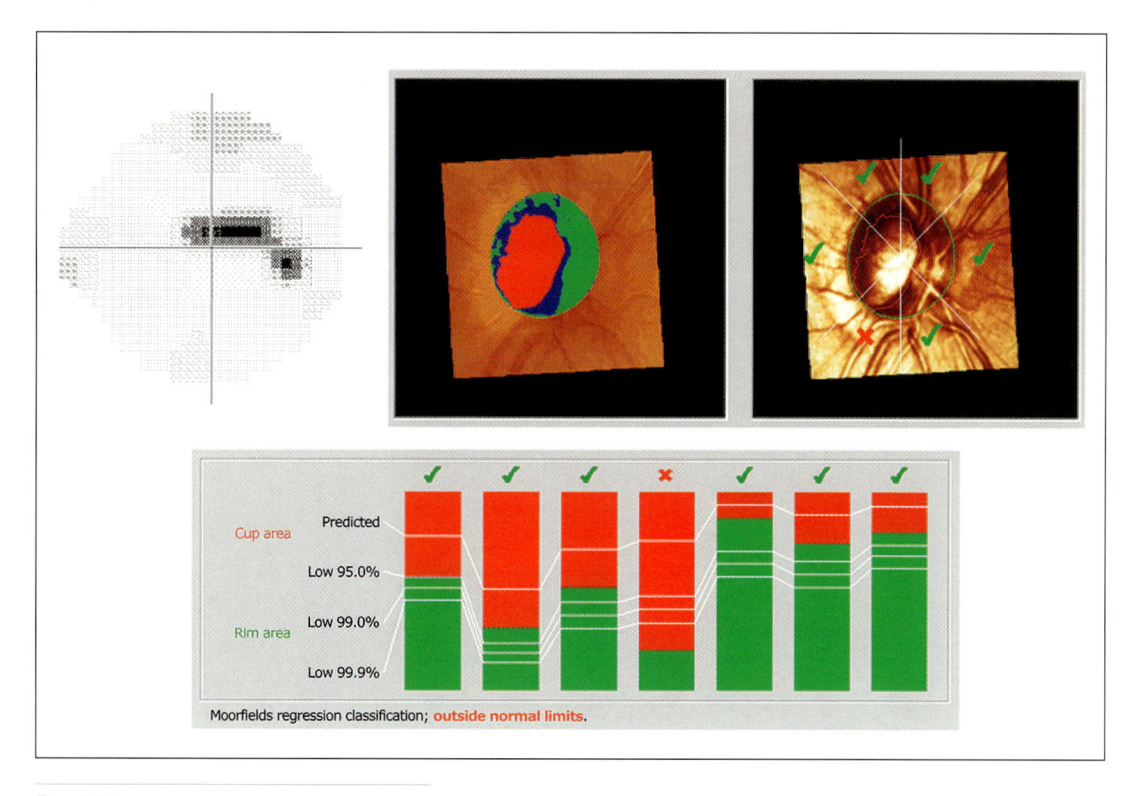

Figure 3.10

Visual field gray scale and HRT II software analysis of an image acquired with the HRT. The infero-temporal segment of the ONH is clearly outside normal limits, and the reflectivity image demonstrates that the loss of the neuroretinal rim is on the temporal side of the infero-temporal segment. This corresponds with the location of visual field loss.

Moorfields Regression Analysis | GARWAY-HEATH

4. Clinical Interpretation of the Heidelberg Retina Tomograph II (HRT II)

Alfonso Antón, MD

Glaucoma causes typical structural changes in the optic nerve head and retinal nerve fiber layer (RNFL). The identification and description of these findings and the detection of changes over time are fundamental components of glaucoma diagnosis and follow-up. The interpretation of findings from the clinical examination of the optic nerve head and RNFL are complex due to the great variability among normal optic disc sizes and shapes, and the presence of other associated diseases. Undoubtedly the most difficult task facing the clinician is longitudinal assessment of the optic disc to establish stability or progression of the disease.

In clinical practice, the evaluation of structural change is usually performed based on fundus biomicroscopy and review of optic disc stereophotographs. Such meticulous assessment at the slit lamp is useful but lacks objectivity and quantification. Optic nerve photographs are objective documents that facilitate comparison of findings over time but require subjective interpretation or color-based computer analysis, and are highly influenced by media opacity or photographic parameters (exposure, light source, digital processing) that may considerably influence the appearance of retinal structures.

Both clinical examination and photographs are part of the standard for glaucoma care. Objective and quantitative measurements of the optic nerve head and RNFL can complement the assessment of glaucomatous damage and can aid in detecting disease progression. The aim of this chapter is to present a systematic approach to the clinical interpretation of HRT II results and to review the usefulness of HRT technology at the time of a single visit.

INTERPRETING THE HRT PRINTOUT

As in any other part of the ophthalmic examination, interpretation of HRT data should be methodical. If it is the first HRT examination for a given patient, the clinician should carefully review the single-test printout. The following is a step-by-step approach to the interpretation of the printout.

1. Check image quality by noting the mean topography standard deviation (SD) at the bottom of the list of stereometric parameters. Review focus, clarity, and centration of the optic nerve head and consider any written comments documenting difficulties that may have occurred during image acquisition. Quality increases as SD value decreases (it is good under 30 µm and, if possible, it should not be over 40 µm). If the SD is greater than 40 µm, the test should be repeated to improve reproducibility or the results should be interpreted with caution.

2. Review the position of the contour line. Use both the reflectance and the topography images to place the contour line at the inner margin of the scleral ring. Sometimes it may be easier to place it on a single tomography image from the image series. HRT parameters are calculated based on the location of the contour line, so the results may vary dependent upon its placement. However, it is important to remember that once positioned on the baseline image, it will be imported to all subsequent images and parameters will change relative to the baseline result. If difficulty is encountered positioning the contour line, placing it marginally outside the scleral ring (i.e., greater than the optic nerve head boundary) is preferable to placing the contour line within the disc itself. Results incorporating small proportions of parapapillary retina give parameters that more accurately reflect the characteristics of the nerve head than those positioned within the nerve head. The only time this does not hold true is when there is parapapillary atrophy, but in such cases the identification of Elschnig's ring is much easier and unlikely to cause difficulties.

3. Review the left half of the report to learn about the structure of the optic disc. On the topography image, the HRT draws a color-coded map. The red area represents the cup; the blue (sloped) and green (flat) areas represent the neuroretinal rim. These images are very easy to interpret by clinicians since they follow the same drawing principles that are used in clinical charts, and give an overview of the disc. The vertical and horizontal cross-section graphs beside and below the topography image give some idea of the shape of the optic nerve head. Next, look at the list of stereometric parameters. These are more useful at follow-up visits to monitor progression, but disc area, rim area, and cup/disc area ratio can provide relevant information. See below for clarification of the relevance of disc size and how it influences cup/disc ratio.

4. Review the bottom left of the report to note the global classification of either normal, borderline, or outside normal limits. The right half of the page illustrates a sector classification based upon the Moorfields Regression Analysis (see Chapter 3), in which each sector is labeled as normal, borderline, or outside normal limits. This statistical analysis qualifies the relationship between the rim and the cup after comparing patient values with a normative database. At the bottom right of the page a bar graph illustrates this comparison in more detail.

5. Finally, for more detailed information, specific parameter values within the different sectors may be reviewed at the computer screen.

The HRT single-test report should be reviewed methodically. The most important information includes the mean topography SD to assess image quality; the topography map to assess global optic disc anatomy; and the global and sector classification of the Moorfields Regression Analysis.

CLINICAL INTERPRETATION OF HRT RESULTS

This section will review the different applications of HRT data in glaucoma management. The HRT supplies useful, additional clinical information in several ways including quantitative measurements and the detection and location of damage. Quantitative data facilitates comparisons between the two eyes of a single individual and comparison between structural and functional data.

1. Quantitative measures

Optic disc size varies among normal subjects, and ranges between 0.80 and 5.54 mm^2 [1] with differences between ethnic groups.[2] Data from a population-based epidemiological study showed that mean (SD) disc area evaluated with HRT was 2.37 (0.43) mm^2 (range, 1.65 to .13 mm^2), with the smallest disc in this population smaller than the cup of the largest normal disc.[3] In fact, 37.3% of normal optic discs had a linear cup/disc ratio over 0.3.[3] As in routine clinical practice, this large variability present in the normal optic disc can lead to erroneous diagnosis and difficulty in the identification of glaucomatous optic neuropathy. Larger discs typically have larger physiological cups, but the resulting large cup/disc ratio does not necessarily indicate glaucomatous damage. HRT images should be assessed in combination with clinical findings including optic disc size, disc shape, and rim characteristics.

HRT provides one-, two-, or three-dimensional measurements globally and by sector, and compares the results with a normative database. HRT gives precise information about disc area and facilitates the identification of physiologically small discs, within which minimal cupping is expected, or macro discs, where cup/disc ratio may be as high as 0.9 without the presence of glaucomatous damage. A small disc with a large cup/disc ratio is more likely to have glaucoma than an optic nerve with a large disc area (Figures 4.1A, B, C).

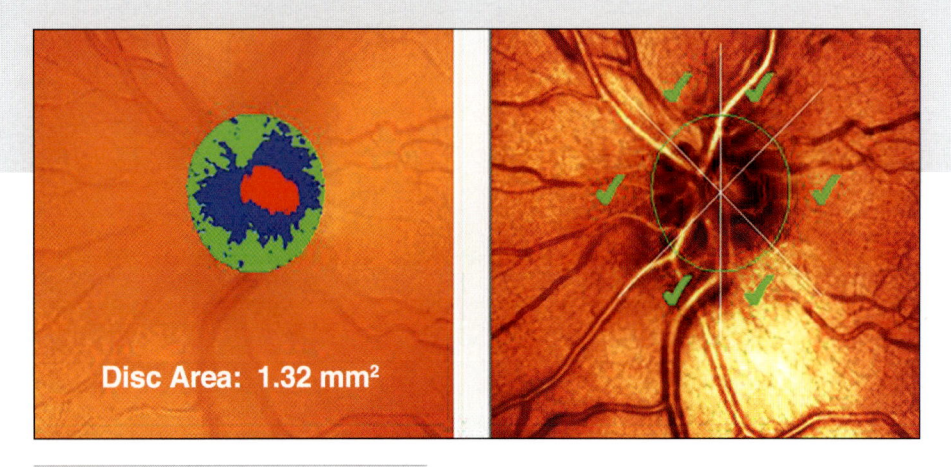

Figure 4.1A
Small normal disc with small cup.

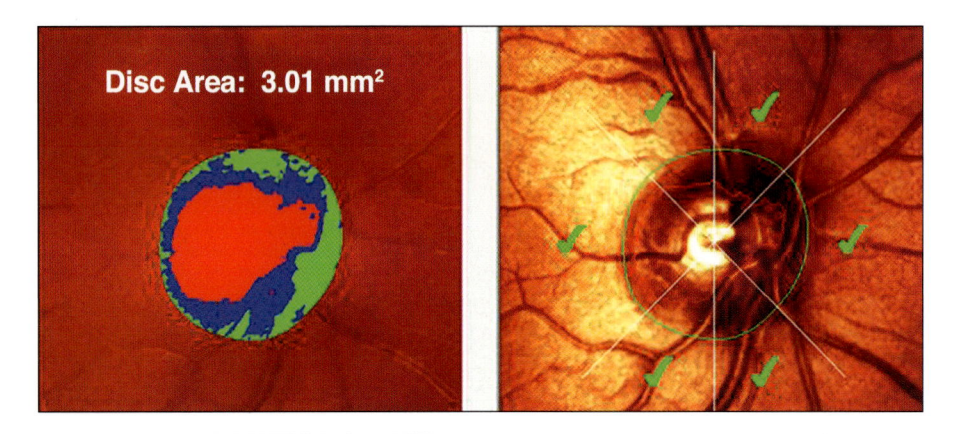

Figure 4.1B
Large normal disc with large physiological cup and cup/disc ratio of approximately 0.7.

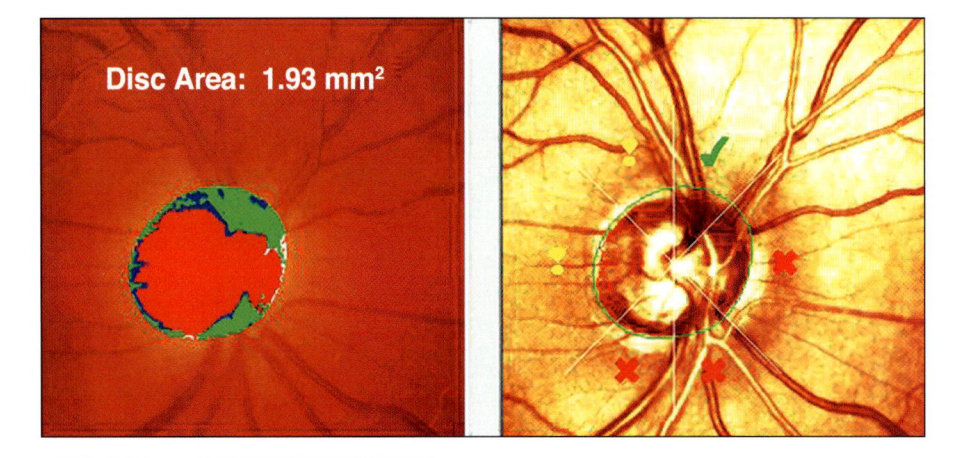

Figure 4.1C
Average size optic disc with large cup/disc due to glaucomatous damage.

44 ANTÓN | Clinical Interpretation of the HRT II

The most constant characteristic of the normal neuroretinal rim, independent of disc size, is the ranked size of the different neuroretinal rim sectors.[1] In most normal eyes the inferior rim is wider than the superior sector, which in turn is wider than the nasal rim, and the temporal rim is usually the narrowest. This rule may be checked with HRT sector data by comparing rim area and/or rim volume in the different sectors. If the inferior rim is narrower than the superior rim, there is probably a loss of nerve fibers in the inferior retina (Figures 4.2A, B).

Quantitative measurements undoubtedly facilitate clinical interpretation of structural damage, but how accurate are HRT measurements? Multiple studies have shown that although HRT, as any other instrument, has certain variability, its measurements are reproducible. The relative height of each pixel or small groups of pixels vary in different measurements, and mean SD ranges from 25 to 49 μm in the worse case.[4-7] Variability is greater in glaucomatous optic nerves than in normal optic nerves (Table 4.1).

HRT measurements are reproducible and show mean SD of 25 to 49 μm for relative height values and 0.04 to 0.06 mm² for rim or cup area. This reproducibility is certainly unreachable by any estimation performed at the slit lamp by an experienced clinician. Accurate quantitative measurements of the optic disc add useful information to reach clinical decisions.

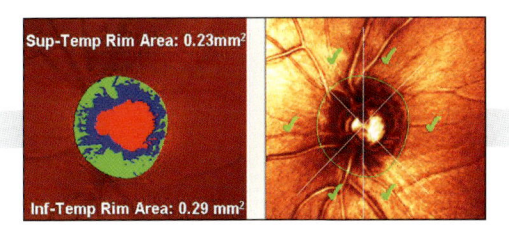

Figure 4.2A
Normal eye with inferior rim sector larger than superior rim sector.

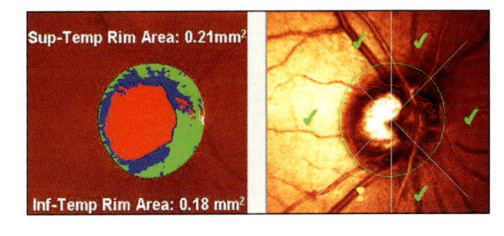

Figure 4.2B
In this eye with initial glaucomatous damage, inferior rim sector is smaller than superior rim, indicating loss of nerve fibers in the inferior rim.

TABLE 4.1

	Method	AUTHOR	NORMAL	GLAUCOMA
MSD	Pixel by pixel	Dreher	38-42	41-49
MSD Equivalent	64 x 64 pixels	Chauhan	25	31
MSD Equivalent	10 x 10 pixels	Cioffi	25	
MSD	Pixel by pixel	Weinreb	30	31

Reproducibility of HRT measurements. Mean standard deviation (MSD) of HRT relative height measurements (μm) as evaluated in different studies.[4-7]

2. Detection of damage

Moorfields Regression Analysis[8] is able to identify structural damage by comparing patient data to a normative database of Caucasian eyes with refractive error under 6 diopters and disc size between 1.2 and 2.8 mm². It evaluates the neuroretinal rim area to disc area ratio globally and at each of six sectors. Individual values are classified as within normal limits if they are inside the 95% confidence interval for normality (green check), borderline if between 95% and 99.9% (yellow exclamation mark), and outside normal limits if outside the 99.9% confidence interval (red X). (Moorfields Regression Analysis is described in detail in Chapter 3).

Many studies have evaluated HRT as a diagnostic tool for glaucoma.[9-12] Table 4.2 summarizes the results of some of these studies and demonstrates that HRT is able to classify normal and glaucoma eyes with accuracy at least as good as stereoscopic photographs evaluated by an experienced glaucoma specialist. Indeed, at the recent consensus meeting of the Association of International Glaucoma Societies on Structure and Function in the Management of Glaucoma, it was agreed that "sensitivity and specificity of imaging instruments for detection of glaucoma are comparable to that of expert interpretation of stereo colour-photography and should be considered when such expert advice is not available." Caution is recommended when evaluating very small or very large optic discs due to the limited normative database and the intrinsic difficulty to assess those eyes. Iester et al[13] found that both sensitivity and specificity of HRT tend to be lower in unusually small discs.

Abnormal HRT results suggest the presence of objective structural damage, but HRT data should never be considered alone. HRT results should be assessed as part of a patient's clinical history and examination, and need to be interpreted together with other clinical findings. HRT adds information and supports clinical decisions but does not substitute clinical examination or assessment of functional damage.

TABLE 4.2

AUTHOR	YEAR	SENSITIVITY	SPECIFICITY
Mikelberg	1995	87	84
Iester	1997	74	88
Uchida	1996	77-92	86-93
Caprioli	1998	85	81
Bathija	1998	78	87
Wollstein	1998	84	97

Diagnostic accuracy of HRT for the diagnosis of glaucoma.[9-12] The algorithm implemented in HRT II was developed and tested by Wollstein et al.[8]

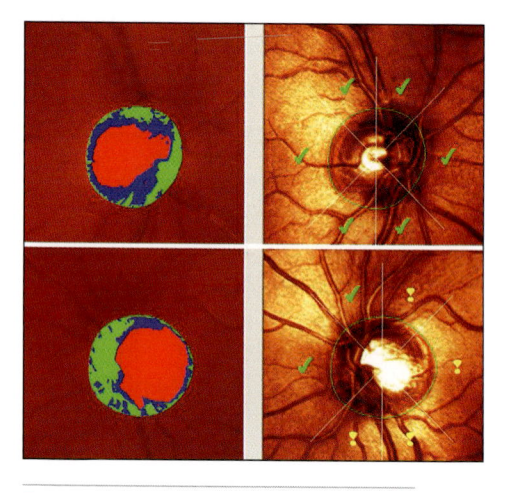

Figure 4.3

HRT images of a 36-year-old woman with pigment dispersion syndrome, intraocular pressures of 26-28 mm Hg, normal and reliable standard visual fields, large discs (3.1-3.3 mm²), and large cups. HRT is able to detect early inferior and temporal rim thinning in the left eye.

An example of how HRT data can help in clinical decision making is shown in Figure 4.3. It shows the HRT images of a 36-year-old woman with pigment dispersion syndrome, intraocular pressures of 26 to 28 mm Hg, normal and reliable standard visual fields, and large discs with no clear signs of rim thinning observed during clinical examination. HRT was able to detect early inferior rim thinning in the left eye and helped establish the diagnosis of early glaucomatous optic neuropathy.

3. Location of damage

Sector analysis is useful to locate structural damage of the rim. Use the upper right graph (reflectance image with Moorfields Regression Analysis) for this purpose. Glaucoma may affect any sector of the disc, but the disease tends to alter inferior-temporal and/or superior-temporal regions earlier than nasal or temporal sectors. HRT helps to locate and describe axonal loss as focal or diffuse. Figures 4.4A & B shows two cases of focal inferior damage, and Figures 4.4C & D show two cases of diffuse damage.

4. Comparison between eyes

It is useful to compare both eyes to interpret clinical findings. Most people have small differences in disc size and shape between eyes, and substantial cup/disc ratio asymmetry is considered suspicious of glaucoma. Nevertheless, epidemiological studies have shown that cup/disc asymmetry is more frequent than initially expected in normal eyes. The Blue Mountains Eye Study found cup/disc asymmetry over 0.2 in 6% of the normal population.[14] Cup/disc asymmetry is most likely to be physiological if there is also a proportional size asymmetry—that is, if the larger disc also has the higher cup/disc ratio. On the contrary, a cup/disc asymmetry between two eyes with the same disc area suggests the presence of axonal loss and acquired enlargement of the cup (Figures 4.5A, B).

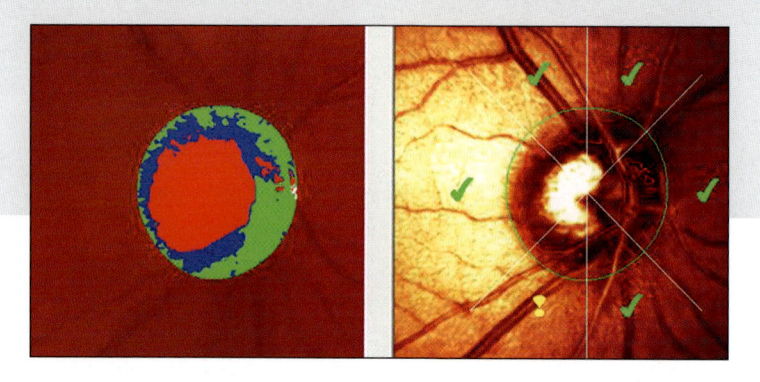

Figure 4.4A
Initial rim thinning.

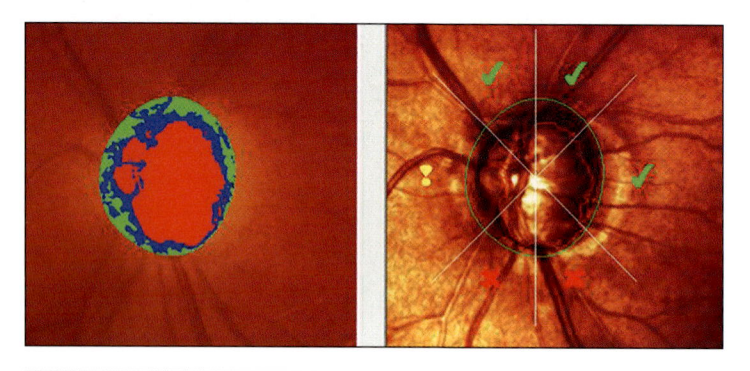

Figure 4.4B
Relatively moderate inferior rim damage in a fairly large disc.

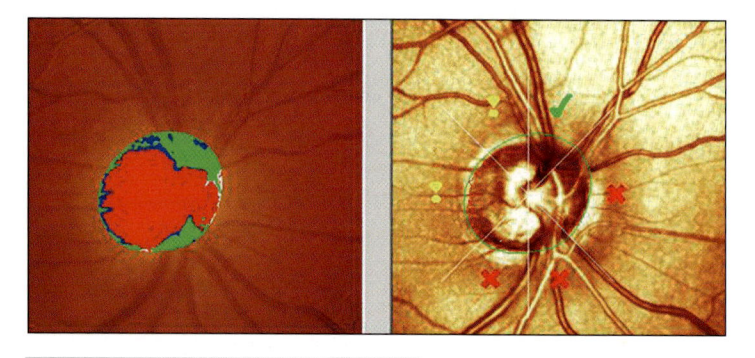

Figure 4.4C
Advanced glaucoma with superior and inferior rim loss.

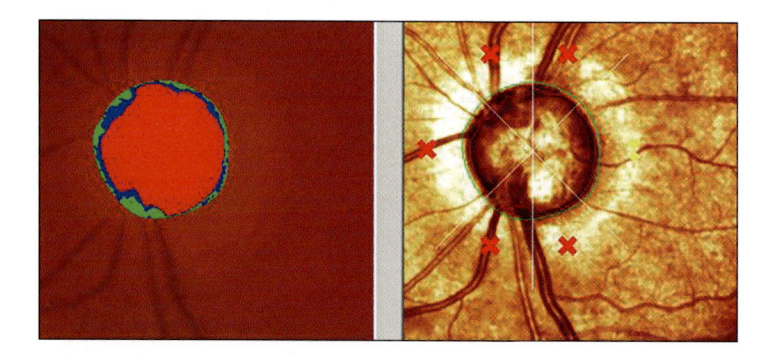

Figure 4.4D
End-stage glaucoma with extensive diffuse loss.

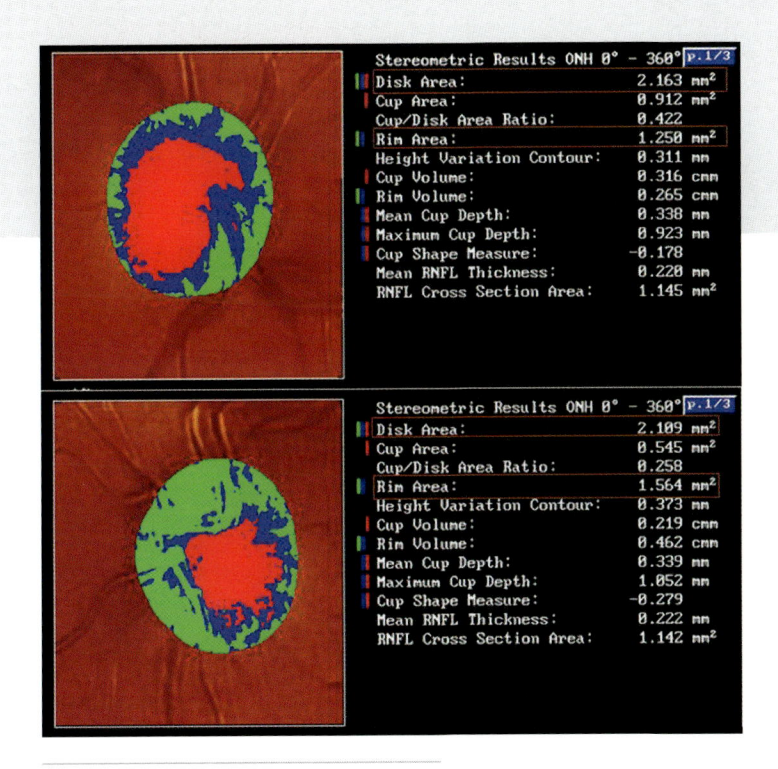

Figure 4.5A

Cup/disc asymmetry with symmetric disc area. There is temporal and inferior rim thinning due to glaucoma in the right eye.

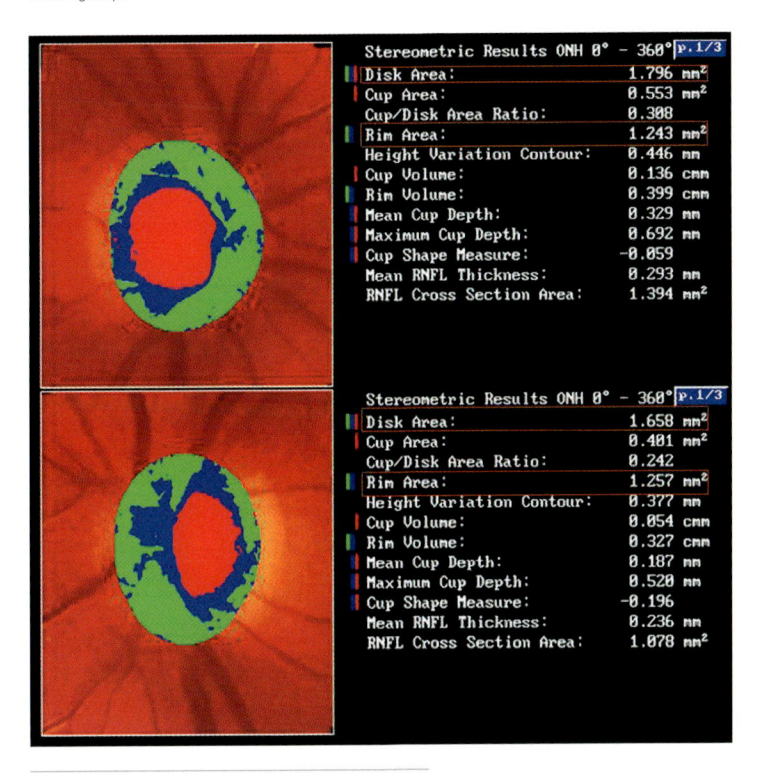

Figure 4.5B

Normal eyes with cup/disc asymmetry but simultaneous disc area asymmetry. Rim area is 1.2 mm² in both eyes, and no signs of glaucomatous damage are present.

5. Comparison of structural and functional damage

There is a relationship between degree and location of functional and structural damage in glaucoma.

Structural damage typically precedes detectable functional damage, so it is relatively common to find structural changes and a normal achromatic visual field. In general, structural and functional changes correlate well along the course of glaucoma although they don't necessarily run parallel, and comparison of the degree of optic nerve and visual field deficits is dependent on the sensitivity of the individual test used. HRT has shown the ability to detect damage in cases with early glaucomatous field loss.[9, 10] In some cases, as shown in Figure 4.3, HRT may detect rim thinning before it is apparent on functional tests.[15] Sector analysis offers the chance to compare the location of structural damage to the location of the functional deficit. When the location of optic nerve defect doesn't match that of visual field defect, the diagnosis should be questioned. Inferior rim parameters correlate well with superior hemifield indices and vice versa, and, although considerable variability is present, the relation between optic nerve and field defects tends to follow certain topographical patterns.[16] Inferior rim thinning is usually associated with superior field defects (Figure 4.6). Nasal visual field defects adjacent to the horizontal meridian match with rim damaged areas close to the vertical midline; rim thinning is usually temporal in the superior hemiretina and affects both sides of the vertical meridian in the inferior retina. Central and paracentral field defects are associated with rim thinning located temporal from the vertical midline, and more peripheral field defects match with the inferior and superior nasal sectors.[16] Therefore, one should always look for correspondence between rim defects and visual field scotomas.

6. Follow-up

The most difficult task of optic nerve assessment is longitudinal assessment to establish stability or progression of the disease. Algorithms to detect progression or change have been improved in the HRT II and are described elsewhere (see Chapter 5). Initial longitudinal data by Chauhan et al[17] indicate the HRT is particularly useful for monitoring progression in glaucoma.

CONCLUSION

In summary, HRT offers a quick and easy method of obtaining quantitative optic nerve data. It complements clinical examination and assessment of visual function in the diagnosis of glaucoma, glaucoma suspects, or ocular hypertension. Clinicians should evaluate the HRT printout looking to answer the classic questions: Is the optic disc normal? Are the discs of both eyes symmetrical? Is there rim thinning or notching? Where is it? Is there enlarging of the cup? Do structural changes match with functional deficits? Is the patient stable or progressing? Finally, the data should always be interpreted in the context of clinical history, examination findings, and other test results.

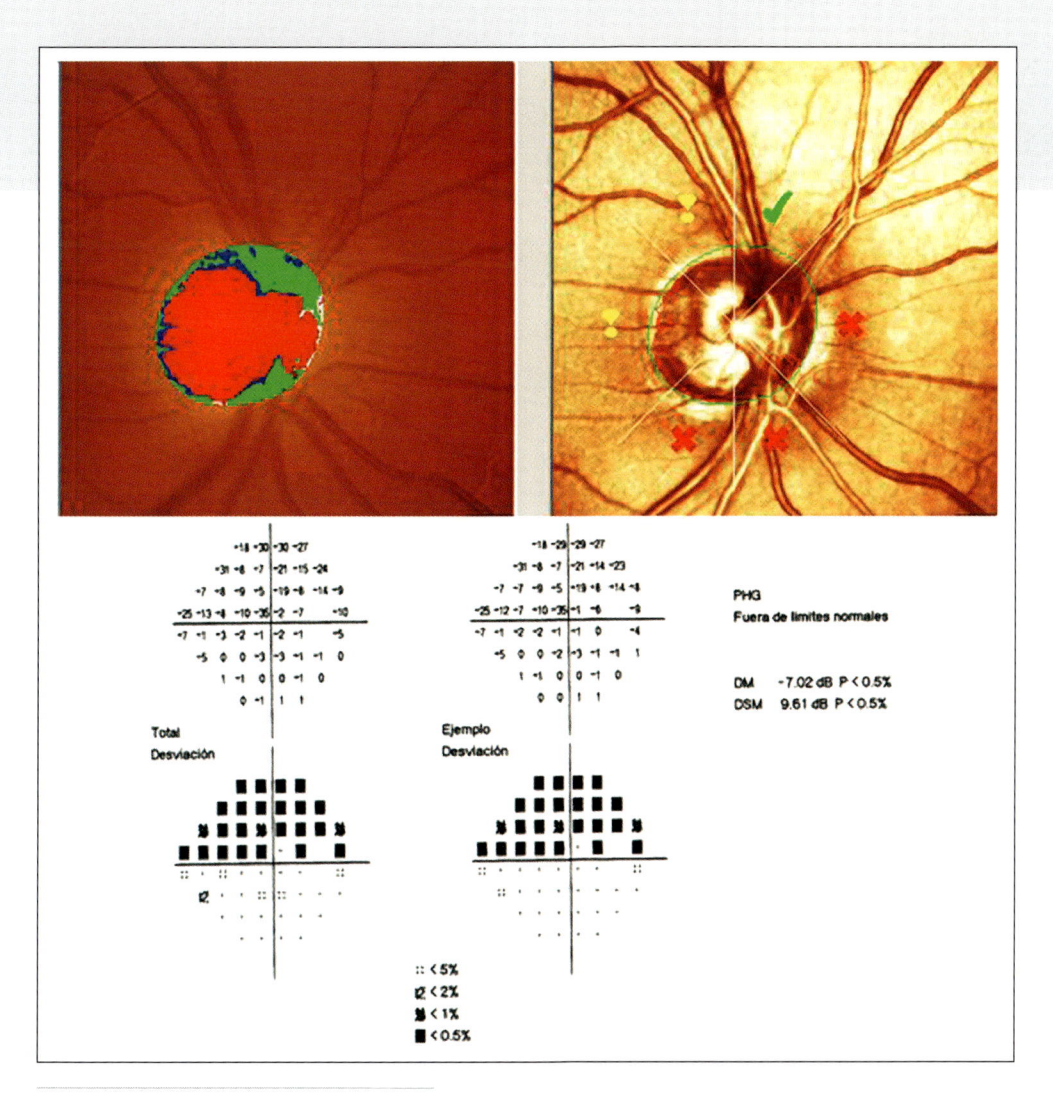

Figure 4.6
Inferior rim thinning associated with superior visual field defect.

REFERENCES

1. Jonas JB, Gusek GC, Naumann GO. Optic disc, cup and neuroretinal rim size, configuration and correlations in normal eyes. *Invest Ophthalmol Vis Sci.* 1988;29:1151-1158.

2. Chi T, Ritch R, Stickler D, Pitman B, Tsai C, Hsieh FY. Racial differences in optic nerve head parameters. *Arch Ophthalmol.* 1989;107:836-839.

3. Anton A, Andrada MT, Aguilera A, Calle MA. Characteristics of the normal optic disc in a Spanish population. *Invest Ophthalmol Vis Sci.* 2000;41:S286.

4. Dreher AW, Weinreb RN. Accuracy of topographic measurements in a model eye with the laser tomographic scanner. *Invest Ophthalmol Vis Sci.* 1991;32:2992-2996.

5. Chauhan BC, LeBlanc RP, McCormick TA, Rogers JB. Test-retest variability of topographic measurements with confocal scanning laser tomography in patients with glaucoma and control subjects. *Am J Ophthalmol.* 1994;118:9-15.

6. Cioffi GA, Robin AL, Eastman RD, Perell HF, Sarfarazi FA, Kelman SE. Reproducibility of optic nerve head topographic measurements with the confocal laser scanning ophthalmoscope. *Ophthalmology.* 1993;100:57-62.

7. Weinreb RN, Lusky M, Bartsch DU, Morsman D. Effect of repetitive imaging on topographic measurements of the optic nerve head. *Arch Ophthalmol.* 1993;111:636-638.

8. Wollstein G, Garway-Heath DF, Hitchings RA. Identification of early glaucoma cases with the scanning laser ophthalmoscope. *Ophthalmology.* 1998;105:1557-1563.

9. Mikelberg FS, Parfitt CM, Swindale NV, Graham SL, Drance SM, Gosine R. Ability of the Heidelberg Retina Tomograph to detect early glaucomatous visual field loss. *J Glaucoma.* 1995;4:242-247.

10. Uchida H, Brigatti L, Caprioli J. Detection of structural damage from glaucoma with confocal laser image analysis. *Invest Ophthalmol Vis Sci.* 1996;37:2393-2401.

11. Caprioli J, Park HJ, Ugurlu S, Hoffman D. Slope of the peripapillary nerve fiber layer surface in glaucoma. *Invest Ophthalmol Vis Sci.* 1998;39:2321-2328.

12. Bathija R, Zangwill L, Berry CC, Sample PA, Weinreb RN. Detection of early glaucomatous structural damage with confocal scanning laser tomography. *J Glaucoma.* 1998;7:121-127.

13. Iester M, Mikelberg FS, Drance SM. The effect of optic disc size on diagnostic precision with the Heidelberg Retina Tomograph. *Ophthalmology.* 1997;104:545-548.

14. Ong LS, Mitchell P, Healey PR, Cumming RG. Asymmetry in optic disc parameters: the Blue Mountains Eye Study. *Invest Ophthalmol Vis Sci.* 1999;40:849-857.

15. Mardin CY, Horn FK, Jonas JB, Budde WM. Preperimetric glaucoma diagnosis by confocal scanning laser tomography of the optic disc. *Br J Ophthalmol.* 1999;83:299-304.

16. Anton A, Yamagishi N, Zangwill L, Sample PA, Weinreb RN. Mapping structural to functional damage in glaucoma with standard automated perimetry and confocal scanning laser ophthalmoscopy. *Am J Ophthalmol.* 1998;125:436-446.

17. Chauhan BC, McCormick TA, Nicolela MT, LeBlanc RP. Optic disc and visual field changes in a prospective longitudinal study of patients with glaucoma: comparison of scanning laser tomography with conventional perimetry and optic disc photography. *Arch Ophthalmol.* 2001;119:1492-1499.

5. Detection of Glaucomatous Changes in the Optic Disc

Balwantray C. Chauhan, PhD

INTRODUCTION

The role of any imaging device for the optic disc in glaucoma is to determine the likelihood of a disc being abnormal and whether the appearance of the disc has changed over a period of time.

The ability to objectively and correctly detect a normal or glaucomatous disc using a single examination depends on the overlap of the distribution of some quantitative measure (such as cup/disc ratio) in unselected glaucoma and normal populations. If the distribution of cup/disc ratios in this population of glaucoma subjects overlaps widely with that of nonglaucomatous subjects, then the utility of this parameter is limited. If, on the other hand, another parameter were to separate the glaucomatous and nonglaucomatous populations into two distinct groups, then the utility of this parameter is likely to be high.

Detection of change depends largely on the ability of an imaging device to detect a meaningful difference that is over and above the measurement variability in a given optic disc. For example, if the variability of measurements of a disc parameter is so large that it encompasses the true change that can occur in a progressing disc, then its utility is likely to be limited. On the other hand, if the measurement variability is low, then small changes may be detected.

IMPORTANCE OF DETECTING OPTIC DISC CHANGES

Detecting optic disc progression is one of the most important aspects of glaucoma management. Accurate and early detection of disc change allows the clinician to make appropriate clinical decisions and, if necessary, monitor and adjust the patients' treatment regimen.

It should be noted that detection of early disc change can be used for making a diagnostic decision. As mentioned above, the inter-individual variation in optic disc parameters is considerable, and many individuals who are not glaucomatous may be classified as glaucomatous. More importantly, individuals who are in the statistically normal range may undergo optic disc change over time and still remain within the normal range when analyses of single examinations alone are done. For example, a patient with an initial cup/disc ratio of 0.5 in a large disc may have a concentric enlargement of the cup such that the cup/disc ratio is now 0.6. While the disc has clearly changed, analyses based on single examinations would classify the disc as normal on both occasions. Hence, in such situations, the fact that the disc has changed may be used as a diagnostic cue that the patient is abnormal and, depending on other clinical factors, an early diagnosis of glaucoma may be made on the strength of the disc change.

The availability of serial optic disc images is a powerful clinical tool in the management of glaucoma (Figure 5.1). The ability to perform sophisticated analysis online provides the clinician with important information that has not been available until now.

OPTIONS FOR DETECTING OPTIC DISC CHANGE

Summary indices

Clinicians are familiar with classical indices of optic disc morphology such as cup/disc ratio, cup volume, and neuroretinal rim area. These summary indices are clinically intuitive and convenient to use. Modern imaging devices such as the Heidelberg Retina Tomograph (HRT) automatically calculate stereometric parameters after a contour line demarking the optic disc has been drawn. When a series of images over time have been obtained and carefully aligned, any change in these parameters can be examined by comparing the values from any follow-up examination to the baseline. If many images are available, a trend analysis that examines whether the change is statistically significant over time (and, more importantly, the rate of change over time) can be calculated.

Optic disc changes usually occur in a non-uniform manner across the disc—that is, progression may be more rapid in some disc sectors compared to others. For this reason, it is useful to divide the disc into sectors in which the summary parameters can be analyzed over time. In this manner, changes in, say, the temporal sector alone become more obvious than in a global analysis in that variability or noise from measurements in the other sectors that are not changing can mask the localized changes in the temporal sector.

INDIVIDUAL TOPOGRAPHIC VALUES

The HRT and the HRT II provide a rich matrix of topographic height values (256 × 256 and 384 × 384 pixels respectively) for each single or mean image. An alternative or additional approach to using the summary measures is to examine the height changes in these individual values to determine whether there has been a change. Because analysis of many thousands of values has to be made, care must be taken during both the statistical analysis and interpretation of the results.

The advantage of this approach is that it places no reliance on a contour line or reference plane. Furthermore, the analysis can be performed over the whole image and not restricted to the optic disc.

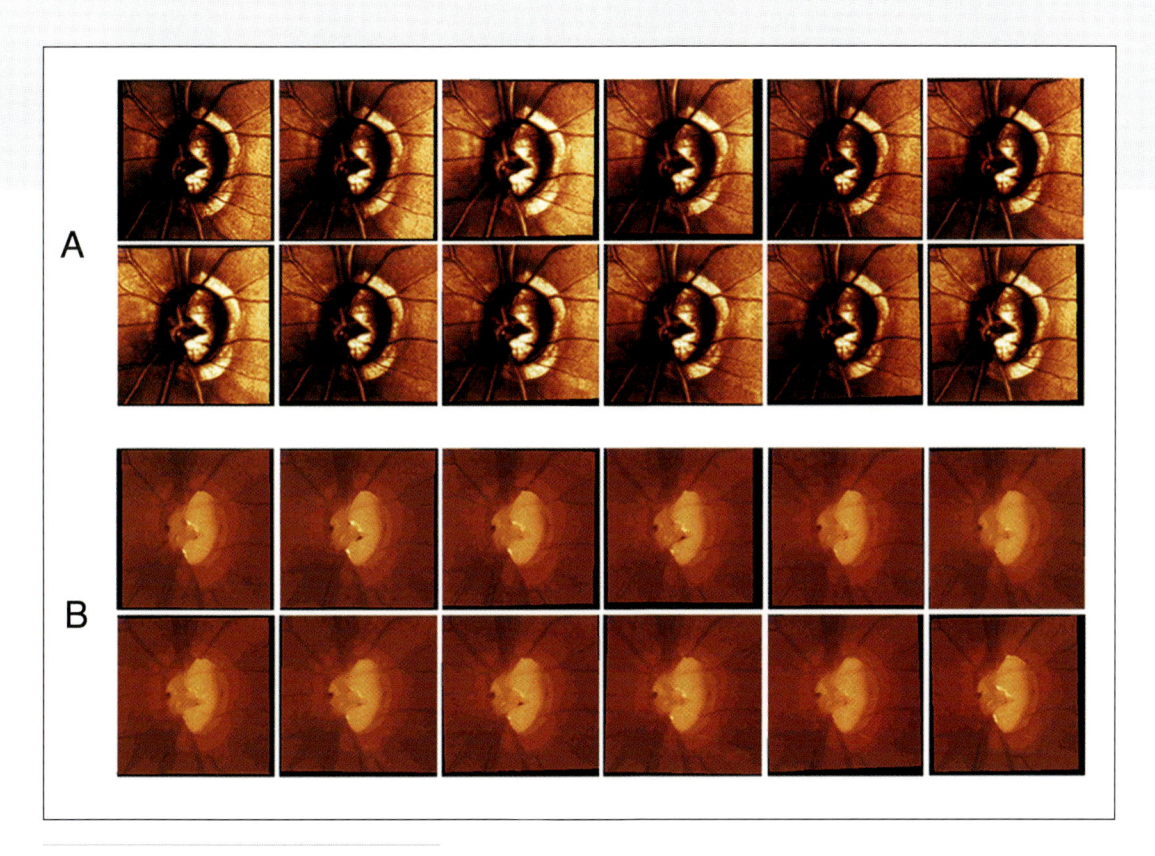

Figure 5.1

HRT images from a four-year follow-up of the left eye of a glaucoma patient examined every four months.

A. Reflectivity images from the series beginning with the baseline image (September 1999, top left) and ending with the final image (October 2003, bottom right).

B. Topography images from the series (baseline [top left] to final [bottom right]).

ANALYSIS OF THE STEREOMETRIC PARAMETERS

The HRT computes a variety of stereometric summary parameters, which have been described in previous chapters. When there are sufficient examinations in the follow-up, the parameters, either singly or in combination, can be observed over time. The number of examinations required before this analysis can be performed depends on the degree of change observed. In cases where large and rapid changes in the optic disc have occurred, quantitative analysis may be possible in as few as three or four examinations, while in cases where the variability of the images is high and/or the changes are small, a larger number of examinations would be required. Generally, as is the case in all types of diagnostic tests, the higher the number of examinations, the better the confidence with the data can be used clinically.

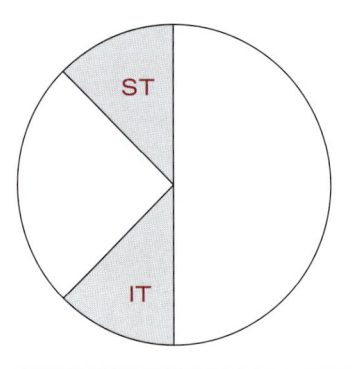

Figure 5.2A
Superior temporal (ST) and inferior temporal (IT) segments, with each segment subtending 45°.

DIVISION OF DISC SECTORS FOR ANALYSIS

The HRT software allows three types of division of disc sectors (Figures 5.2A, B, C) for analysis of the parameters over time (Figures 5.3A, B). In the first, analysis can be done in the superior temporal and inferior temporal sectors; in the second, in the superior and inferior sectors; and in the third, in the entire upper or entire lower disc. In each case, analysis of the entire or global value or values is also performed.

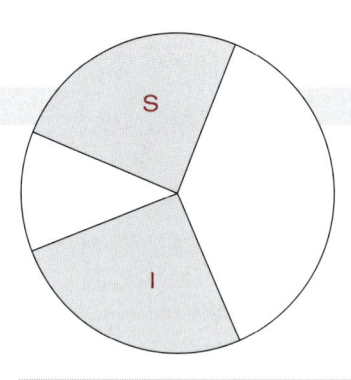

Figure 5.2B
Superior (S) and inferior (I) segments, with each segment subtending 90°.

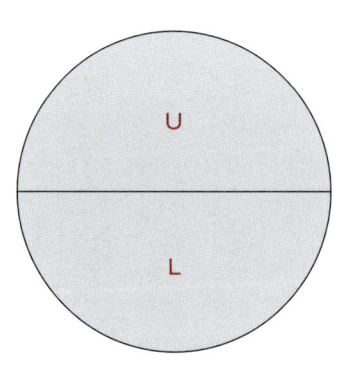

Figure 5.2C
Upper (U) and lower (L) segments, with each segment subtending 180°. Format for the right eye is shown.

ANALYSIS AND INTERPRETATION OF THE PARAMETERS

When performing a trend analysis, the following parameters can be examined over time:

1. Rim area
2. Rim volume
3. Cup volume
4. Cup shape
5. Mean retinal nerve fiber layer thickness
6. Mean height of contour
7. Mean contour elevation
8. Contour line modulation temporal
9. Mean cup depth
10. Mean height inside contour line
11. A combination or average of the above parameters

The actual values of the parameters are not shown in the trend analysis, but instead the normalized change from baseline is shown (Figures 5.3A, B). The normalization is done in order to place the change from baseline in all parameters on the same scale from +1 (maximum improvement) to −1 (maximum deterioration). The basis of the normalization is a ratio of (the difference between a given value and baseline) to (the difference between the average value in a normal eye and an advanced glaucomatous eye).

The horizontal axis can be displayed on a real-time scale with examination dates or simply by examination number irrespective of the time interval between examinations. A formal regression analysis is not performed; therefore, the user should adopt empirical rules for the interpretation of change. Previous experience has shown that a downward trend in three consecutive examinations is suggestive of change; however, confirmations in further examinations are always very useful.

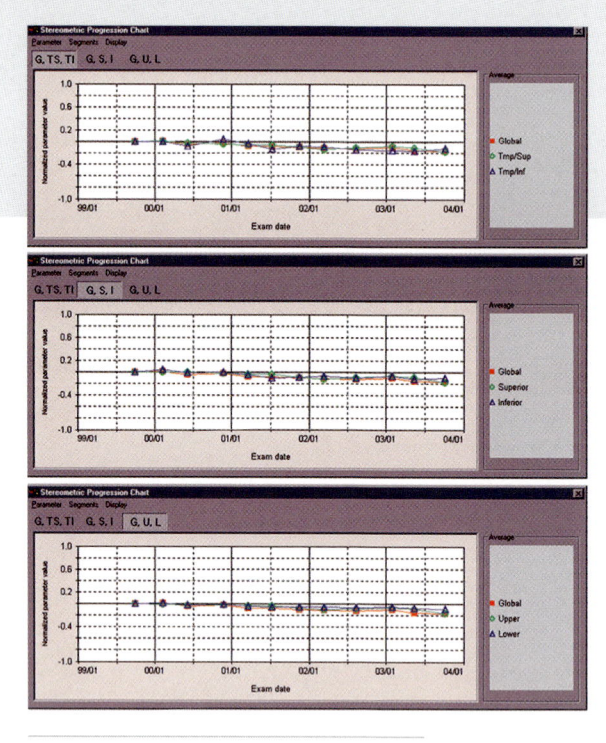

Figure 5.3A

Trend analysis of the parameters of the follow-up shown in Figure 5.1. Analysis of the average of the 10 parameters with the three divisions of disc sectors (top to bottom respectively) as shown in Figures 5.2A, B, C.

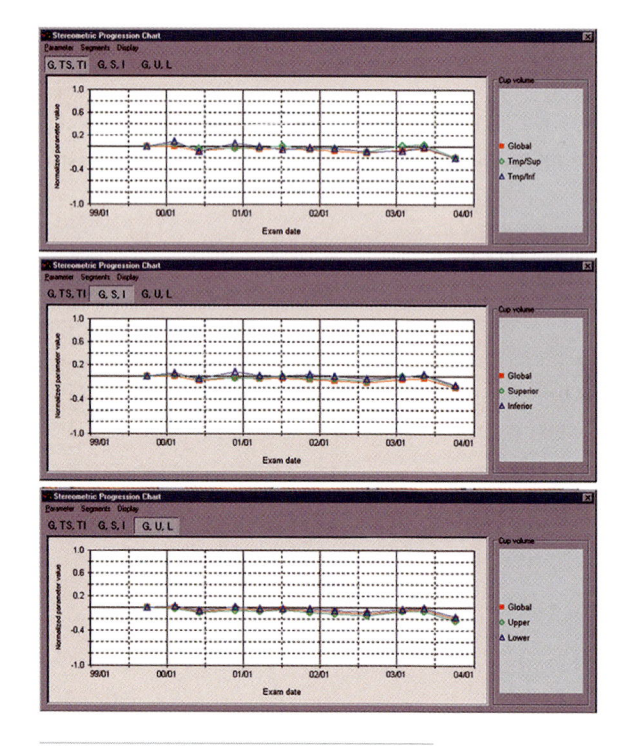

Figure 5.3B

Respective analysis of cup volume. The analysis of the average of the parameters shows a very subtle but definite trend toward worsening values, which is not apparent in the analysis of cup volume.

TOPOGRAPHIC CHANGE ANALYSIS

Topographic change analysis (TCA) is a statistical method to compare the topographic values in discrete areas of the image called superpixels, which contain 4 x 4 (or 16 pixels) at two points in time.[1] Typically, after a series over time has been obtained and aligned, comparison of each follow-up image is made to the baseline.

There are many differences between the trend analysis previously described and TCA, the most important being that TCA does not require a contour line or a reference plane. The analysis is performed on the raw topography values. TCA computes, at each superpixel, the probability of the difference in height values between the two time points occurring by chance alone. Hence, a high probability value (when p is high) indicates that the likelihood of a change is low. On the other hand, a low probability (when $p < 0.05$) indicates that there is little chance that the difference was due to chance alone and that the change was likely to be real. The key determinant in TCA is the variability in topography values within the superpixel over the two sets of three images for each comparison. If the local variability is high, a much larger height difference between the two time points will be required to reach statistical significance, and vice versa. Typically the variability of measurements is highest at the edge of the optic cup and along blood vessels, and lowest in the topographically flatter peripapillary retina. Therefore, relatively larger changes will be required to reach significance in the former case and relatively smaller changes in the latter.

TCA DISPLAY

TCA is automatically performed (Figure 5.4) when there is one mean baseline image and at least two mean follow-up images, with each mean containing at least three individual images.

The main analysis from TCA is contained in the Change Probability Maps, which show each of the follow-up images either in a single display showing each of the reflectivity or topography images (Figure 5.5) or individually (Figure 5.6). In the individual Change Probability Map it is possible to display the baseline reflectivity or topography image as well as the respective follow-up images, in addition to the gray scale of the p values from the analysis and the Absolute Change Map (Figure 5.6). The Reflectivity Map is overlaid with red and green symbols that show superpixels in which the p values are significant, with red demonstrating depression and green demonstrating elevation (Figures 5.5 and 5.6). It is important to note that, by default, only those superpixels where the p values are significant over three consecutive examinations are shown. It is highly recommended that this option ("3 consecutives" as opposed to "2 consecutives") is used.

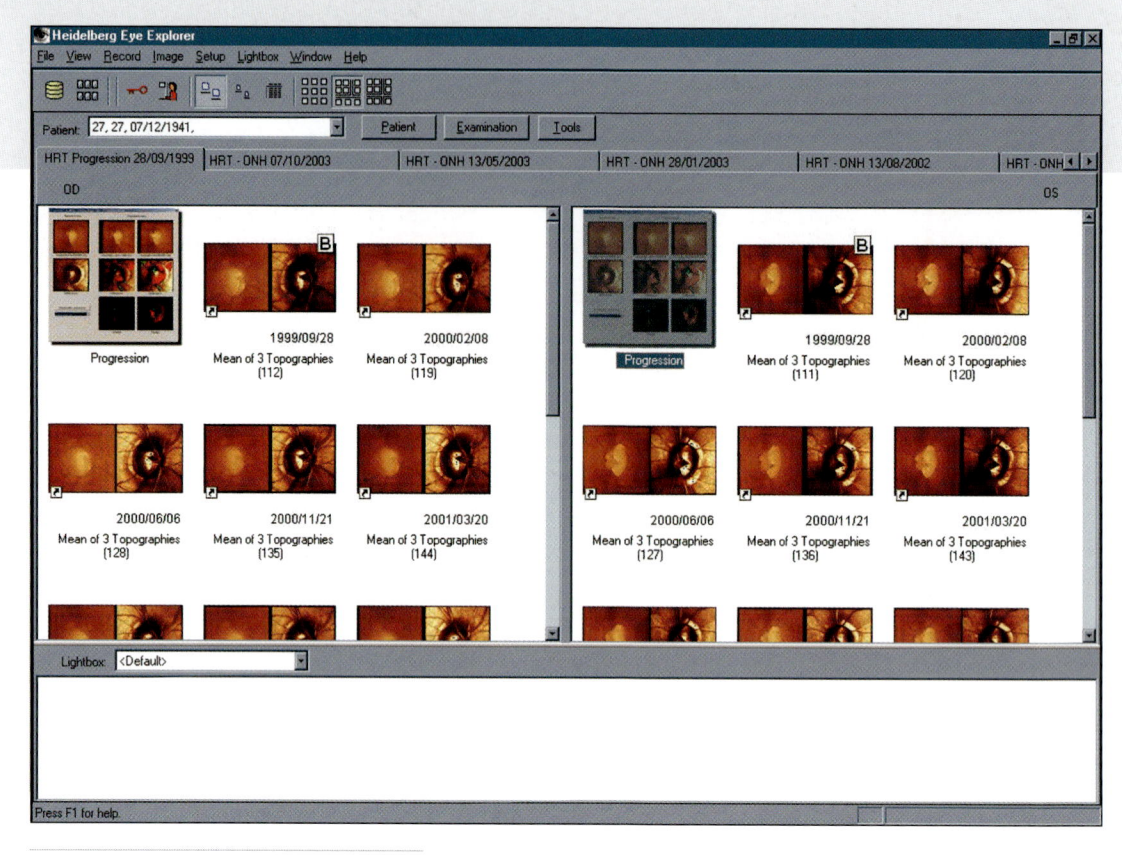

Figure 5.4

A window from the HRT software showing the examinations in the follow-up of each eye in addition to the Progression icon to initiate TCA and trend analysis.

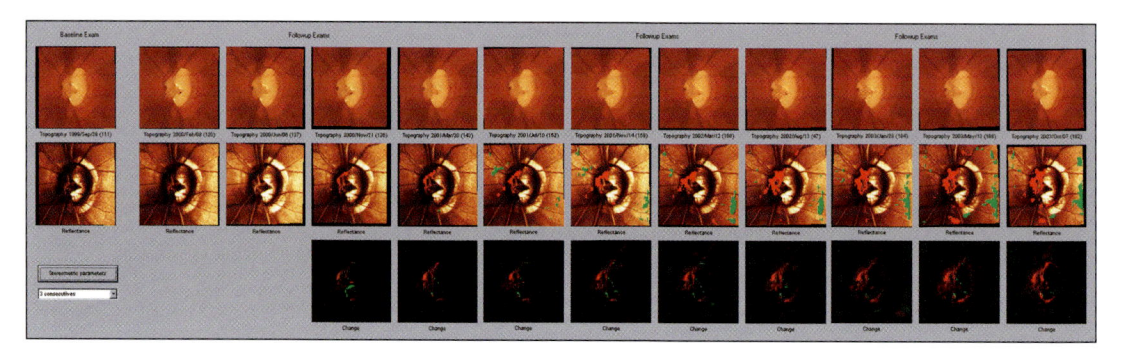

Figure 5.5

Initial window from TCA showing the serial topography images (top), the reflectivity images with the superimposed red and green probability symbols showing areas of depression and elevation respectively (middle), and the absolute difference (from baseline) images color-coded such that the redder or greener the superpixels, the greater the depression or elevation respectively (bottom). This disc shows clear change both supero-nasally and inferiorly (see probability and difference maps). While there are significant green superpixels, they are limited mostly to the edge of the image, where there are likely some alignment errors. The change in these locations is also very small (bottom). Finally, the changes in this disc are more evident with TCA than in the trend analysis (Figure 5.3A) or in inspection of the reflectivity or topography images (Figure 5.1).

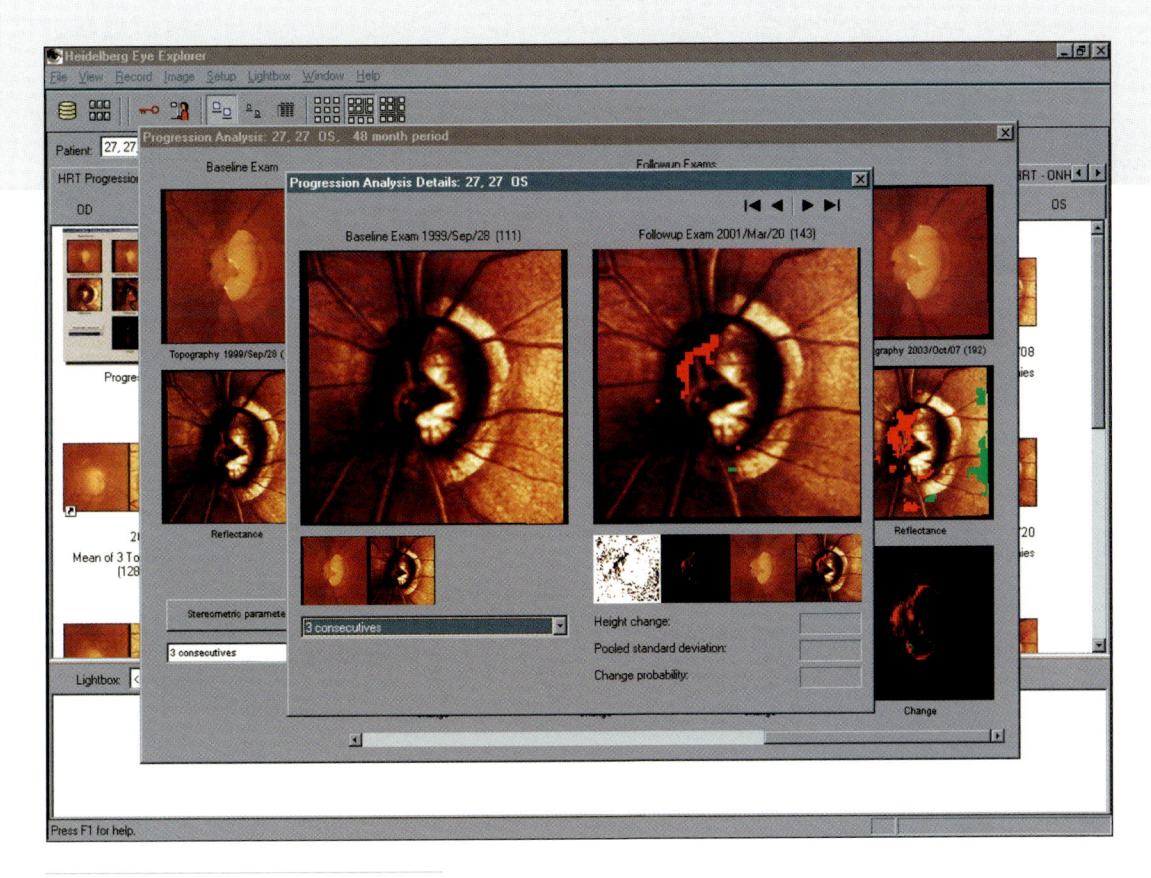

Figure 5.6

Window from TCA after mouse-clicking on any of the follow-up reflectivity images. In addition to the disc change supero-nasally compared to baseline, the nerve fiber layer defect infero-temporally appears more pronounced. The user can toggle between the baseline reflectivity and topography images by mouse-clicking on the respective thumbnail image under the main window and also between the follow-up Raw Probability Map, Absolute Change Map, topography, and reflectivity respectively by mouse-clicking on the respective thumbnail image under the main window.

The user can determine the change in local areas by mouse-clicking any area on the follow-up image to reveal the change, pooled standard deviation, and p value in that superpixel (Figure 5.7).

INTERPRETATION OF TCA

TCA is a powerful analysis that has been demonstrated to detect very small changes in optic disc and peripapillary retinal topography. There are, however, no rules regarding when the change detected becomes clinically significant. In a recent study,[2] the criterion for significant change was the presence of a cluster of 20 superpixels derived from cutoff values obtained as the 95th percentile in a group of normal subjects followed over time. It is very important to distinguish between criteria for progression in research studies and in individual patients in a clinical setting. In the latter situation, the criteria may be different for different patients depending on the individual risk.

TCA is a statistical analysis and therefore while a given amount of change in one patient may be highly significant, in another it may not reach significance for a variety of reasons. Even though findings are significant, one should examine the magnitude of change to determine whether the rate or amount of change is meaningful. On the other hand, the absolute change or rate of change in another patient may be high; however, due to variability, the change may not reach statistical significance. These changes cannot be entirely disregarded, and efforts should be made to ensure that the variability of the images is the lowest it can be. Unfortunately, to date, there are no proven guidelines on what degree or rate of change in absolute units (i.e., μm or μm per year) is clinically significant principally because we do not have an external or gold standard for progression.

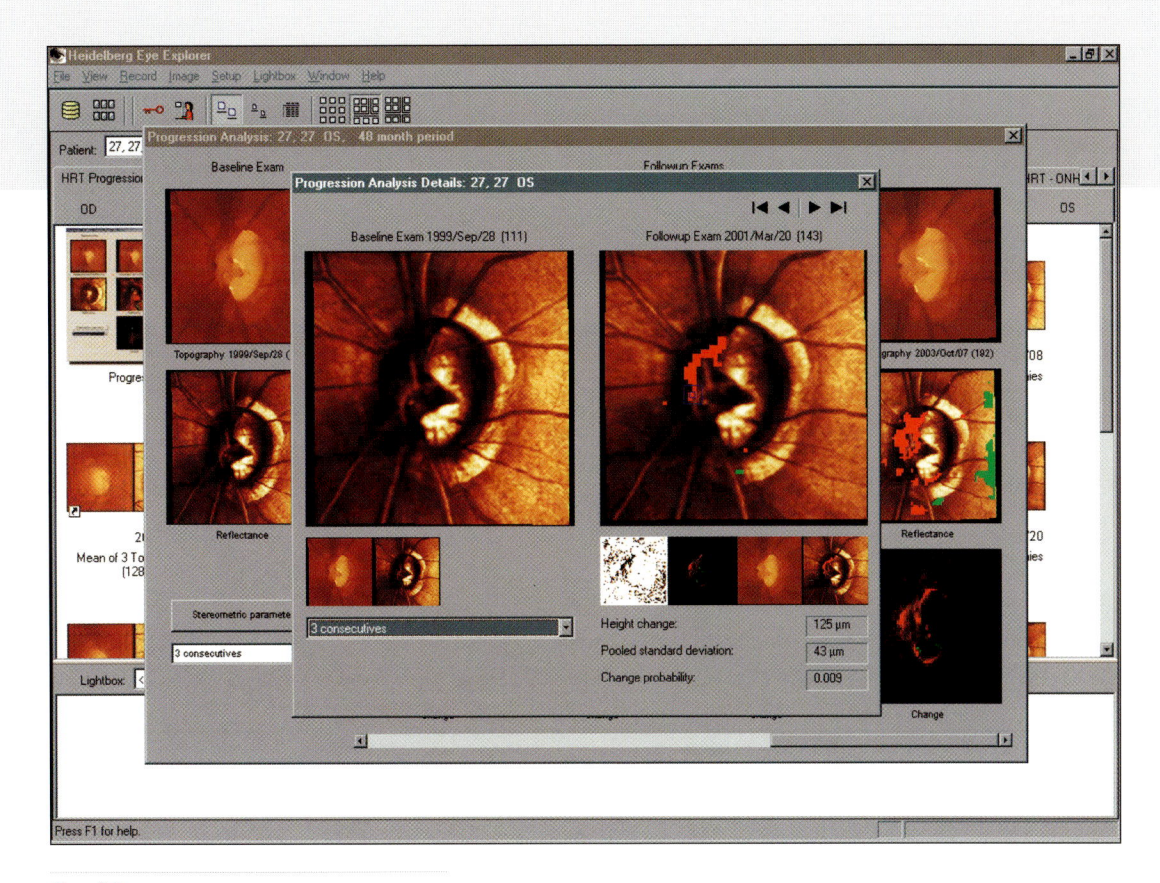

Figure 5.7

Window from TCA after mouse-clicking anywhere on the follow-up reflectivity image. The outer blue square contains 4 X 4 (16) superpixels or 16 X 16 (256) pixels. The center blue square contains one superpixel. The height change, pooled standard deviation (of the six constituent values), and the p value in that superpixel are shown in the bottom right of the window.

PRACTICAL ISSUES AND TIPS FOR USING THE HRT TO DETECT CHANGE

Image acquisition

- Image quality is paramount. Remember that garbage in = garbage out.

- Ensure that the utmost care is taken to obtain the best possible quality images. Do not rush the acquisition process and if in doubt obtain more images than necessary. Only the best quality images can then be used in the analysis and the others discarded. This is much easier than asking the patient to return to the clinic in case the only set of images obtained was unsatisfactory.

- During image acquisition ensure that the:
  - Patient is given a fixation target if the internal fixation target is difficult to see and/or if the disc cannot be centered in the image frame (see below).
  - Laserbeam enters through the center of the pupil.
  - Fundus is illuminated as evenly as possible.
  - Optic disc is in the center of the image frame. This is crucial for follow-up because it ensures that there is maximum overlap in the area of the aligned images and also that the reference ring (different from the reference plane), which is used to align the serial images, is well away from the disc edge.
  - Optic disc is well enclosed within the image frame with at least 0.5 disc diameters of peripapillary retina visible. If not, switch to a wider scan angle (HRT only, since the scan angle with the HRT II is fixed to 15°).

- Before computing the mean topography, ensure that there are no significant eye movements (especially slow drift or pursuit movements). Use the "Show movie" option of the image series.

- When performing an analysis of the parameters or using TCA, ensure that the serial images are properly aligned. This can be done by mouse-clicking the control buttons on the top right of the screen (Figure 5.6) and cycling between the images. If there are obvious alignment errors, specific images can be removed from the series and/or the manual alignment method should be used. Remember, good alignment of serial images is critical for TCA to perform optimally. Poor alignment will also affect the analysis of parameters.

FREQUENCY OF EXAMINATIONS

- Generally, the more images during the follow-up, the better the analysis. Having a large number of examinations also allows the removal of obviously poor ones for the analysis. This has less of an impact on any change analysis if there are many examinations available in the first place.

- Because examinations are relatively quick, they should ideally be performed routinely in the same way that intraocular pressure or visual acuity is measured.

- Obtain a good set of baseline images (up to three sets). Usually the image quality at baseline is more variable or poorer in quality. Having more images means that the user is not limited to one set.

- When change is suspected, more examinations should be performed over a shorter period of time. In this way the TCA can be used in a shorter time period.

INTERPRETATION

- The greatest utility of the HRT is in the detection of change. Detection of change can be used both for the diagnosis of glaucoma and progression of disc damage.

- Examine all the results carefully. Remember, the quality and options offered by the software are much better than the printout. Always examine the results on the computer monitor and never rely on the printout alone.

- Obtain as many high-quality images as possible.

- Be judicious about excluding images of poor quality and alignment. The inclusion of these images often leads to erroneous results.

- Many patients show changes with the HRT. While this change is not normal, it does not always mean there is clinically significant progression. On the other hand, if there are other signs of disc progression (determined by clinical examination or disc photographs), do not assume the HRT is correct. There are potential reasons why the HRT may miss optic disc change.

- In clinical care, the HRT is a powerful tool that should be used with other clinical tools and measures. In the final analysis, machines do not replace sound clinical judgment.

REFERENCES

1. Chauhan BC, Blanchard JW, Hamilton DC, LeBlanc RP. Technique for detecting serial topographic changes in the optic disc and peripapillary retina using scanning laser tomography. *Invest Ophthalmol Vis Sci.* 2000;41:775-782.

2. Chauhan BC, McCormick TA, Nicolela MT, LeBlanc RP. Optic disc and visual field changes in a prospective longitudinal study of patients with glaucoma: comparison of scanning laser tomography with conventional perimetry and optic disc photography. *Arch Ophthalmol.* 2001;119:1492-1499.

6 Structural/Functional Relationships in Glaucoma

George A. Cioffi, MD, and Chris A. Johnson, PhD

HISTORY OF STRUCTURE / FUNCTION RELATIONSHIPS IN GLAUCOMA

The relationship of the structural integrity of the optic nerve and the functional status of the visual system has been actively investigated since the invention of the direct ophthalmoscope more than 150 years ago. The ability to assess both the structure and function of the optic nerve has evolved, becoming more clinically practical and efficient with greater sensitivity and specificity for detection of disease. However, the evolution of structural and function diagnostics have not always developed in concert. As visual field documentation has become more sensitive and more precise, we have increasingly used functional testing for diagnosis and monitoring of the glaucomatous optic nerve. Over the last century and a half, there have been many advances in functional detection of disease and assessment of progression. Clinicians have relied on the most efficient, sensitive, and specific test method (functional or structural) that was available at any given time. Therefore, even if a structural change is antecedent to a functional change, sensitive functional testing has developed more quickly and been implemented to a greater extent into clinical practice. Yet even von Graefe hinted at the relationship of visual field documentation and optic nerve changes.[1] Further illumination regarding the relationship between the appearance of the optic nerve and visual field deficits associated with glaucoma were founded through the pioneering efforts of Jaeger, Weber, Mackenzie, and others.[2]

In addition to exploiting the best available testing paradigms of any particular era, the recent understanding that measurable functional and structural changes of optic nerve may not occur simultaneously has once again forced us to rethink the structure-function relationship. The understanding that early in the disease structural optic nerve alterations may be more easily observed has led to intense interest in objective optic nerve analysis. While late in the course of the disease, functional changes may be a better barometer of optic nerve health. However, functional tests have continually improved, becoming more sensitive to early change and narrowing the gap between observable functional loss and its precedent structural alteration. This chapter will review the history of the structure-function relationship and discuss the various diagnostic tests that have been used to evaluate the glaucomatous optic nerve. In addition, recent longitudinal studies that shed more light on the relationship between structure and function will be reviewed.

Over the last 40 years, a number of investigators reported a strong relationship between the appearance of the optic nerve and retinal nerve fiber layer and visual field deficits in patients with glaucoma.[3-11] Drance[3-5] reported that he was correctly able to determine whether an eye had glaucomatous visual field loss on the basis of the appearance of the optic nerve with 85% sensitivity and 80% specificity. Other studies have reported similar results.[12,13] In addition, several investigators have also reported that changes in the optic nerve head precede visual field loss.[14-17] Susanna and Drance[18] conducted a prospective, longitudinal study of the false positives and true negatives of predicting the visual field status on the basis of optic nerve appearance. This investigation suggested that, in some cases, there were early optic nerve changes that preceded visual field loss. Hart et al[15] and Gloster[19] reported an increase in the prevalence of glaucomatous visual field loss with increasing cup/disc ratios. In addition, Hart et al[15] also reported that high cup/disc ratios strongly correlated with later development of visual field loss. Taken together, these studies provided strong evidence that optic nerve structural anomalies were highly correlated with visual function deficits.

In recent decades, more investigations have examined the relationship between clinically observable structural abnormalities of the optic disc and perimetric changes. These investigations have focused on a variety of different features of the optic nerve and the surrounding nerve fiber layer. In addition, localized topographic changes have been associated with regional functional changes. Holmin[20] evaluated the ability of readers to classify a quadrant of the optic nerve in disc photographs and predict whether a visual field deficit was present. Good agreement was found among the readers, who demonstrated 75% sensitivity and 85% specificity for predicting visual field loss in the superior and inferior hemifields on the basis of optic disc appearance. Lewis et al[21] examined the ability to predict early, moderate, and advanced glaucomatous visual field loss from the appearance of the optic disc in primary open-angle glaucoma and low-tension glaucoma. The severity of visual field loss could be accurately predicted about 50% of the time. Overprediction and underprediction of visual field loss occurred approximately equally, although there were large individual differences among observers.

Several investigators have also reported strong correlations between neuroretinal rim thickness and visual field deficits, both for overall measures and for localized regions.[22-28] Weber et al[29] found good topographic correlations in patients with focal optic nerve damage between the affected region of the neuroretinal rim of the optic nerve and visual field deficits. Neuroretinal rim thickness, either average rim thickness or localized rim thickness, appears to be the most consistent optic disc parameter to correlate with visual field measures across a large number of investigations.

Although longitudinal investigations of structural and functional losses in glaucoma are not common, those that have been published indicate that structural changes of the optic disc or retinal nerve fiber layer usually occur prior to visual field loss as determined by conventional white-on-white perimetry.[27,30-35]

Historically, it has been generally believed that structural abnormalities of the optic nerve and retinal nerve fiber layer precede visual function loss, particularly using standard automated perimetry. However, the advent of new visual function test procedures that are more sensitive than standard automated perimetry (SAP) opens the possibility that some visual function deficits may be concurrent with or prior to observable structural glaucomatous damage. Presently, optic nerve head analysis is also rapidly evolving, and more sensitive techniques have become available. This will presumably allow earlier detection of glaucomatous structural changes, permitting observable structural change to predate functional consequences. To date, no prospective longitudinal investigations have directly compared the temporal relationship of structural and functional glaucomatous changes for the new, more sensitive visual function test procedures and more advanced structural analysis methods.

OPTIC NERVE IMAGE ANALYSIS AND FUNCTIONAL LOSS

A number of investigations have evaluated the relationship between optic nerve parameters determined using objective image analysis and visual fields. Caprioli and Miller[36] found significant correlations for cup/disc ratio, disc rim area, and cup volume (Rodenstock Scanning Laser Ophthalmoscope) and visual field indices (mean defect and loss variance). Using the Heidelberg Retina Tomograph (HRT), Brigatti and Caprioli[37] found even stronger correlations between optic disc parameters and visual field indices. In particular, the correlation of the third central moment of the frequency distribution of depth values (cup shape) with both mean deviation and corrected pattern standard deviation were quite high. Lee et al[38] examined the relationship between HRT optic nerve measurements and visual field indices. Rim area, rim volume, and mean retinal nerve fiber layer height were all significantly correlated with both mean deviation and corrected pattern standard deviation. The cup shape was also significantly correlated with mean deviation. The highest correlation was between rim area and mean deviation. There was also a strong correlation between rim area of the superior and inferior sections of the optic nerve and the corresponding visual field hemifields.

Iester and colleagues[39, 40] also reported good correlations between HRT optic nerve parameters and visual field indices. Rim area was found to be the best optic nerve predictor of mean deviation. In addition, they found that superior and inferior optic nerve measures were significantly correlated with visual field indices for the corresponding visual field hemifields. Tole et al[41] also reported significant correlations between HRT optic disc measurements and visual field indices.

Emdadi et al[42] performed HRT measurements in patients with focal glaucomatous visual field loss and conducted a quantitative comparison of the topography of optic disc characteristics with the focal visual field deficits. Approximately half of the patients demonstrated diffuse optic disc damage despite having a focal visual field defect. About 25% to 35% of patients had focal optic nerve deficits, and about 15% had no detectable optic disc deficit. These findings suggest that distinct topographic relationships between optic disc damage and visual field loss are not always strongly correlated. However, in a subsequent study of patients with both focal optic disc damage and focal visual field loss[43] a strong relationship was found between damaged optic disc sectors and the location of visual field loss. Kamal et al[44] evaluated a small group of ocular hypertensive patients who had converted to glaucomatous visual field loss in comparison to a small group of normal control eyes. Significant optic disc changes were noted in the ocular hypertensives converting to glaucoma. In addition, the HRT optic disc changes were noted prior to the development of confirmed visual field change.

Several investigators have examined the relationship between quantitative optic disc measurements obtained with a confocal scanning laser ophthalmoscope and short-wavelength automated perimetry (SWAP) and motion sensitivity. Yamagishi et al[45] evaluated the relationship between focal optic disc damage as determined by Heidelberg Retina Tomograph images, and localized visual field deficits for SWAP in glaucoma. There was a strong topographic relationship between the SWAP visual field deficits and damaged nerve rim sectors. In addition, Teesalu and colleagues[46,47] compared SWAP visual field sensitivity to several optic disc parameters and retinal nerve fiber layer height obtained from the Heidelberg Retina Tomograph. They found high correlations for SWAP visual field indices and hemifield values in comparison to several optic disc parameters (cup shape measure, rim volume, rim area) and retinal nerve fiber layer measures (retinal nerve fiber layer height and retinal nerve fiber layer cross-sectional area).

The topographic relationship between motion perimetry deficits and optic disc abnormalities was examined by Bosworth et al[48] in patients with focal optic nerve damage and focal motion perimetry losses. Comparisons were also made to SWAP and standard automated perimetry deficits. A strong topographic relationship was observed between optic disc abnormalities and motion perimetry deficits. These topographic correlations were also found for standard automated perimetry and SWAP. Thus, focal notching of the optic nerve is probably independent of specific subsets of retinal ganglion cells because all three visual function tests showed similar topographic relationships to the optic nerve and each visual function test is believed to be mediated by different groups of retinal ganglion cells.

Although these investigations all report strong relationships between focal functional deficits and focal optic nerve deficits, it should be kept in mind that a large proportion of glaucomatous optic nerve damage is characterized by diffuse thinning of the neuroretinal rim, where topographic structure/function relationships are not expected to be as strong.

CRITERIA FOR ASSESSING VISUAL FUNCTION LOSS IN GLAUCOMA

In an effort to better understand the relationship between structure and function, it should be realized that assessing loss, either structural or functional, involves a number of investigator-driven choices. These choices or criteria have evolved over several decades for automated perimetry and are presently being developed for automated optic nerve head analysis. The Structure and Function Evaluation (SAFE) study was a prospective, collaborative investigation of a large population of ocular hypertensives, glaucoma suspects, and early glaucoma patients.[10] To date, there have been two publications from the SAFE study. The first manuscript described the development of a system or set of criteria for determination of visual field loss in ocular hypertension and early glaucoma. The findings indicated that it is possible to derive criteria with high specificity for detecting the development of early glaucomatous visual field loss that can be applied to both SAP and SWAP results. Both the evaluation of individual visual field locations and analyses based on nerve fiber bundle patterns appear to have the best overall performance. Specificities of 98% to 100% were achieved by using these analyses in conjunction with requiring all potential changes to be confirmed on two successive visual field examinations. Previous investigations have also found that to maintain high specificity, it is necessary to confirm suspected changes with additional examinations.[49] These findings indicate that it is possible to attain high specificity with confirmation on two successive visual field examinations. However, most of the SAFE results were based on the evaluation of ocular hypertensive patients, who have lower test-retest variability than glaucoma patients. Clustered abnormal points provided a slight improvement in specificity, but nothing that was as significant as confirmed abnormalities.

Six criteria were found to have high specificity, and of these six, two of them (GHT [glaucoma hemifield test] outside normal limits and four pattern deviation locations that were worse than the 5% probability level) had the highest percentage of abnormal results detected for SAP. The GHT outside normal limits also detected a higher number of new SWAP deficits. The establishment of these criteria for the development of glaucomatous visual field loss allows them to be used in conjunction with analysis of structural features of the optic nerve to determine the relationship between structural and functional losses in glaucoma.

DOES STRUCTURAL CHANGE PREDICT FUTURE FUNCTIONAL DEFICITS?

The second SAFE publication examined the relationship between pre-existing glaucomatous optic neuropathy and the later development of functional abnormalities.[11] The criteria established in the first publication were used to define functional abnormalities. The findings indicated a strong, statistically significant relationship between the presence of glaucomatous optic disc damage at baseline and the subsequent development of SAP visual field loss at some later point in time. The optic nerves were evaluated by masked observers examining simultaneous stereophotographs, obtained at baseline and annually. A similar trend was found for the presence of glaucomatous optic discs at baseline and the presence of SWAP deficits at baseline or development of SWAP deficits during the follow-up period. There were a large number of cases in which the affected visual field hemifield(s) and optic disc hemisector(s) were in correspondence, and an equally large number of cases in which the extent of optic disc damage extended to two hemisectors when the visual field loss was restricted to one hemifield. There were a very small number of cases in which the extent of visual field loss was greater than the degree of optic disc damage.

In addition, in eyes that demonstrated progression of optic disc damage, most developed glaucomatous visual field loss at or subsequent to the time at which the optic disc changes were noted. Taken together, these results provide compelling evidence that visible glaucomatous optic disc changes occur prior to measurable glaucomatous visual field loss, and that glaucomatous optic disc changes are predictive of future visual field loss as measured with current techniques.

In the group that did not demonstrate visual field loss for SAP or SWAP, there were a large number of optic discs that were judged to be glaucomatous. Many of these cases are likely to represent future visual field "conversions" that have not yet manifested themselves during the follow-up interval. A more comprehensive determination of the strength of the relationship between structural and functional damage in glaucoma may require as much as 10 years or more of longitudinal follow-up. Other investigations have concluded that glaucomatous optic disc changes precede visual field loss and that optic disc changes are predictive of future visual field deficits; however, most have been cross-sectional or retrospective. These results from longitudinal monitoring of a large cohort of well-defined patients are consistent with the findings of prior studies and provide strong support for observable structural optic disc abnormalities being a predictor of future glaucomatous visual field deficits. These findings also support the need for standardized and automated optic nerve analysis in the management of glaucoma patients.

CONCLUSION

A large number of studies have demonstrated good correlations between structural alterations of the optic nerve head and retinal nerve fiber layer and visual function deficits produced by glaucoma. Structural and functional glaucomatous damage appears to be topographically related, especially in cases of predominantly focal damage. There is also evidence from prior studies that optic nerve and retinal nerve fiber layer damage usually can be observed prior to visual field loss, at least for standard automated perimetry. Recent investigations indicate that technological advances in both the measurement of structural properties of the optic disc and retinal nerve fiber layer and the evaluation of new visual function characteristics have improved the sensitivity and reliability of noninvasive methods of assessing glaucomatous damage.

There are several shortcomings associated with many investigations of structure/function relationships in glaucoma to date. First, the majority of investigations have involved relatively small numbers of patients. In many instances, inclusion and exclusion criteria are not well defined. Secondly, the vast majority of investigations are cross-sectional. There are very few longitudinal investigations of structure/function relationships, and many of such studies have been conducted retrospectively rather than prospectively. Finally, many of the early studies in particular suffer from methodological flaws, selection biases, and other problems associated with the research design or analysis methods.

Evaluation of a large, prospectively collected data set of functional and structural optic nerve measures in glaucoma patients strengthens the understanding of these issues. There are two fundamental questions to be answered. First, is a structural abnormality predictive of future glaucomatous visual field loss? If so, what is the strength of this relationship? Secondly, what is the relationship between structural optic nerve changes and visual function changes in glaucoma?

In the SAFE study, a strong relationship exists between glaucomatous optic disc damage at study entry and the subsequent development of a confirmed glaucomatous SAP visual field defect. A higher percentage of glaucomatous optic discs were also found in patients with SWAP deficits at baseline and in those who later developed SWAP deficits. These findings support the premise that a glaucomatous optic disc is predictive of the subsequent development of glaucomatous visual field loss.

REFERENCES

1. Traquair HM. *An Introduction to Clinical Perimetry.* St Louis, Mo: Mosby; 1946.
2. Duke-Elder W. Anomalies of the intraocular pressure. In: *Textbook of Ophthalmology,* Vol 3. St Louis, Mo: Mosby; 1941:chap 40.
3. Drance SM. The optic disc and visual field in glaucoma [editorial]. *Can J Ophthalmol.* 1974;9:389-390.
4. Drance SM. Doyne Memorial Lecture, 1975. Correlation of optic nerve and visual field defects in simple glaucoma. *Trans Ophthalmol Soc UK.* 1975;95:288-296.
5. Drance SM. Correlation between optic disc changes and visual field defects in chronic open-angle glaucoma. *Trans Am Acad Ophthalmol Otolaryngol.* 1976;81:224-226.
6. Read RM, Spaeth GL. The practical clinical appraisal of the optic disc in glaucoma: the natural history of cup progression and some specific disc-field correlations. *Trans Am Acad Ophthalmol Otolaryngol.* 1974;78:255-274.
7. Gloster J. Quantitative studies of visual field loss and cupping of the optic disc. Their relevance to the management of chronic simple glaucoma. *Trans Ophthalmol Soc UK.* 1979;99:82-83.
8. Goldberg I. Optic disc and visual field changes in primary open angle glaucoma. *Aust J Ophthalmol.* 1981;9:223-229.
9. Johnson CA, Cioffi GA, Liebmann JR, Sample PA, Zangwill L, Weinreb RN. The relationship between structural and functional alterations in glaucoma: a review. *Semin Ophthalmol.* 2000;15:221-233.
10. Johnson CA, Sample PA, Cioffi GA, Liebmann JR, Weinreb RN. Structure and function evaluation (SAFE): I. Criteria for glaucomatous visual field loss using standard automated perimetry (SAP) and short wavelength automated perimetry (SWAP). *Am J Ophthalmol.* 2002;134:177-185.
11. Johnson CA, Sample PA, Zangwill LM, et al. Structure and function evaluation (SAFE): II. Comparison of optic disc and visual field characteristics. *Am J Ophthalmol.* 2003;135:148-154.
12. Hoskins HD Jr, Gelber EC. Optic disk topography and visual field defects in patients with increased intraocular pressure. *Am J Ophthalmol.* 1975;80:284-290.
13. Hitchings RA, Spaeth GL. The optic disc in glaucoma II: correlation of the appearance of the optic disc with the visual field. *Br J Ophthalmol.* 1977;61:107-113.
14. Drance SM. The disc and the field in glaucoma. *Ophthalmology.* 1978;85:209-214.
15. Hart WM Jr, Yablonski M, Kass MA, Becker B. Quantitative visual field and optic disc correlates early in glaucoma. *Arch Ophthalmol.* 1978;96:2209-2211.
16. Sommer A, Pollack I, Maumenee AE. Optic disc parameters and onset of glaucomatous field loss. I. Methods and progressive changes in disc morphology. *Arch Ophthalmol.* 1979;97:1444-1448.
17. Sommer A, Pollack I, Maumenee AE. Optic disc parameters and onset of glaucomatous field loss. II. Static screening criteria. *Arch Ophthalmol.* 1979;97:1449-1454.
18. Susanna R, Drance SM. Use of discriminant analysis I. Prediction of visual field defects from features of the glaucoma disc. *Arch Ophthalmol.* 1978;96:1568-1570.
19. Gloster J. Quantitative relationship between cupping of the optic disc and visual field loss in chronic simple glaucoma. *Br J Ophthalmol.* 1978;62:665-669.
20. Holmin C. Optic disc evaluation versus the visual field in chronic glaucoma. *Acta Ophthalmol (Copenh).* 1982;60:275-283.
21. Lewis RA, Hayreh SS, Phelps CD. Optic disk and visual field correlations in primary open-angle and low-tension glaucoma. *Am J Ophthalmol.* 1983;96:148-152.
22. Guthauser U, Flammer J, Niesel P. The relationship between the visual field and the optic nerve head in glaucomas. *Graefes Arch Clin Exp Ophthalmol.* 1987;225:129-132.
23. Funk J, Bornscheuer C, Grehn F. Neuroretinal rim area and visual field in glaucoma. *Graefes Arch Clin Exp Ophthalmol.* 1988;226:431-434.
24. Jonas JB, Gusek GC, Naumann GO. Optic disc morphometry in chronic primary open-angle glaucoma. II. Correlation of the intrapapillary morphometric data to visual field indices. *Graefes Arch Clin Exp Ophthalmol.* 1988;226:531-538.
25. Hyung SM, Kim DM, Youn DH. Optic disc and early glaucomatous visual field loss. *Korean J Ophthalmol.* 1990;4:82-91.
26. Nyman K, Tomita G, Raitta C, Kawamura M. Correlation of asymmetry of visual field loss with optic disc topography in normal-tension glaucoma. *Arch Ophthalmol.* 1994;112:349-353.
27. Jonas JB, Grundler AE. Correlation between mean visual field loss and morphometric optic disk variables in the open-angle glaucomas. *Am J Ophthalmol.* 1997;124:488-497.
28. Michelson G, Langhans MJ, Harazny J, Dichtl A. Visual field defect and perfusion of the juxtapapillary retina and the neuroretinal rim area in primary open-angle glaucoma. *Graefes Arch Clin Exp Ophthalmol.* 1998;236:80-85.
29. Weber J, Dannheim F, Dannheim D. The topographical relationship between optic disc and visual field in glaucoma. *Acta Ophthalmol (Copenh).* 1990;68:568-574.
30. Okubo K. Correlation between glaucomatous optic disc and visual field defects. IV. Mode of cupping formation. *Kobe J Med Sci.* 1986;32:197-202.
31. Katz LJ, Spaeth GL, Cantor LB, Poryzees EM, Steinmann WC. Reversible optic disk cupping and visual field improvement in adults with glaucoma. *Am J Ophthalmol.* 1989;107:485-492.
32. Zeyen TG, Raymond M, Caprioli J. Disc and field damage in patients with unilateral visual field loss from primary open-angle glaucoma. *Doc Ophthalmol.* 1992;82:279-286.
33. Zeyen TG, Caprioli J. Progression of disc and field damage in early glaucoma. *Arch Ophthalmol.* 1993;111:62-65.
34. Miglior S, Brigatti L, Lonati C, Rossetti L, Pierrottet C, Orzalesi N. Correlation between the progression of optic disc and visual field changes in glaucoma. *Curr Eye Res.* 1996;15:145-149.
35. Brigatti L, Hoffman D, Caprioli J. Neural networks to identify glaucoma with structural and functional measurements. *Am J Ophthalmol.* 1996;121:511-521.

36. Caprioli J, Miller JM. Correlation of structure and function in glaucoma. Quantitative measurements of disc and field. *Ophthalmology.* 1988;95:723-727.

37. Brigatti L, Caprioli J. Correlation of visual field with scanning confocal laser optic disc measurements in glaucoma [published erratum appears in *Arch Ophthalmol* 1996;114:424]. *Arch Ophthalmol.* 1995;113:1191-1194.

38. Lee KH, Park KH, Kim DM, Youn DH. Relationship between optic nerve head parameters of Heidelberg Retina Tomograph and visual field defects in primary open-angle glaucoma. *Korean J Ophthalmol.* 1996;10:24-28.

39. Iester M, Mikelberg FS, Courtright P, Drance SM. Correlation between the visual field indices and Heidelberg Retina Tomograph parameters. *J Glaucoma.* 1997;6:78-82.

40. Iester M, Swindale NV, Mikelberg FS. Sector-based analysis of optic nerve head shape parameters and visual field indices in healthy and glaucomatous eyes. *J Glaucoma.* 1997;6:370-376.

41. Tole DM, Edwards MP, Davey KG, Menage MJ. The correlation of the visual field with scanning laser ophthalmoscope measurements in glaucoma. *Eye.* 1998;12:686-690.

42. Emdadi A, Zangwill L, Sample PA, Kono Y, Anton A, Weinreb RN. Patterns of optic disk damage in patients with early focal visual field loss. *Am J Ophthalmol.* 1998;126:763-771.

43. Anton A, Yamagishi N, Zangwill L, Sample PA, Weinreb RN. Mapping structural to functional damage in glaucoma with standard automated perimetry and confocal scanning laser ophthalmoscopy. *Am J Ophthalmol.* 1998;125:436-446.

44. Kamal DS, Viswanathan AC, Garway-Heath DF, Hitchings RA, Poinoosawmy D, Bunce C. Detection of optic disc change with the Heidelberg retina tomograph before confirmed visual field change in ocular hypertensives converting to early glaucoma. *Br J Ophthalmol.* 1999;83:290-294.

45. Yamagishi N, Anton A, Sample PA, Zangwill L, Lopez A, Weinreb RN. Mapping structural damage of the optic disk to visual field defect in glaucoma. *Am J Ophthalmol.* 1997;123:667-676.

46. Teesalu P, Vihanninjoki K, Airaksinen PJ, Tuulonen A, Laara E. Correlation of blue-on-yellow visual fields with scanning confocal laser optic disc measurements. *Invest Ophthalmol Vis Sci.* 1997;38:2452-2459.

47. Teesalu P, Vihanninjoki K, Airaksinen PJ, Tuulonen A. Hemifield association between blue-on-yellow visual field and optic nerve head topographic measurements. *Graefes Arch Clin Exp Ophthalmol.* 1998;236:339-345.

48. Bosworth CF, Sample PA, Williams JM, Zangwill L, Lee B, Weinreb RN. Spatial relationship of motion automated perimetry and optic disc topography in patients with glaucomatous optic neuropathy. *J Glaucoma.* 1999;8:281-289.

49. Keltner JL, Johnson CA, Quigg JM, Cello KE, Kass MA, Gordon MO. Confirmation of visual field abnormalities in the Ocular Hypertension Treatment Study. *Arch Ophthalmol.* 2000;118:1187-1194.

7 The Retina Module

John G. Flanagan, PhD, MCOptom and Chris Hudson, PhD

A noninvasive, objective, and quantitative approach to the assessment of retinal edema is both timely and important for the future management of retinal disease, in particular diabetic macular edema.[1-9] It has been predicted that over the next 20 years there will be an unprecedented increase in the prevalence of diabetes and its complications. When this is considered along with the limitations of current clinical standards for the detection of retinal edema, the need for new objective imaging techniques becomes clear. Fundus biomicroscopy and stereophotography both rely upon the subjective evaluation of retinal thickening, which makes it particularly difficult to distinguish the development of retinal edema from normal inter-subject variation[8,10] and detect change in the amount of retinal edema. Even in patients with clinically significant diabetic macular edema, the leading cause of visual impairment in diabetic eye disease, it has been reported that there are dramatic differences between retinal specialists when defining the extent and location of the edema.[8]

The Retina Module of the Heidelberg Retina Tomograph II (HRT II) (Heidelberg Engineering, Heidelberg, Germany) acquires a series of 16 lateral retinal images for every millimeter of scan depth along the axial plane, or z-axis. Once the sections are aligned, the amount of light returned from the eye and falling on the instrument's detector, known as the reflectance intensity, can be plotted for each pixel as a function of scan depth. This plot of reflectance intensity per unit depth is called the confocal intensity profile, or z-profile (Figure 7.1). The standard topographic surface is generated by establishing the position of peak reflectance intensity along the confocal intensity profile for each pixel. This corresponds to the position of greatest refractive index change, i.e., the interface between the vitreous and the internal limiting membrane (for further details see Chapter 1). We previously demonstrated that measuring the width of the confocal intensity profile could provide objective maps of retinal thickening in selected patients with clinically defined macular edema.[6] It was also found that peak reflectance intensity of the profile decreased in areas of edema.[6,7] This was thought to be a result of the reduced change in refractive index found when going between the vitreous and areas of retinal edema. Consequently, an edema index has been proposed that is sensitive to both the increase in signal width and localized change in peak reflectance. The resultant Edema Maps offer a high-resolution image of the extent and magnitude of retinal edema.[7-9,11]

THEORETICAL ASPECTS OF RETINAL EDEMA MAPPING

Edema Maps (EMs) are generated by calculating an edema index (EI) for each pixel location such that:

Edema index$_{x,y}$ = SW$_{x,y}$ / IN$_{x,y}$

where SW$_{x,y}$ is the signal width of the confocal intensity profile at 50% peak reflectance intensity for a given pixel location (x,y) and IN$_{x,y}$ is the peak reflectance intensity for pixel location (x,y) normalized across all image pixel locations (Figure 7.2). The normalization procedure compensates for variation in absolute reflectance intensity between images, caused by eye and head movement, tear film quality, pupil size, and laser/detector alignment.[6, 12] By incorporating two aspects of the effect of edema on the confocal intensity profile, the resultant edema index is sensitive to early retinal edema. The edema index is therefore quantified in arbitrary units.

Signal width (SW$_{x,y}$) is calculated by fitting a 16th order polynomial to the confocal intensity profile and measuring the signal width at 50% of the peak reflectance. The curve-fitting algorithm also enables aspects of quality control. Pixels are considered invalid, appear black in the Edema Map, and are not used in any of the analysis when the polynomial is unable to model the data. This happens with hemorrhage, when much of the signal is absorbed; exudate, when the signal is reflected; and extensive detachment.

IMAGE ACQUISITION

When using the Retina Module it is essential that care and attention is given to the process of image acquisition and that the image quality is optimal. In particular it is important that the image is appropriately focused and that the brightness across the image is even, with attention being given to the corners of the live image prior to acquisition. Each of these steps in the acquisition process are similar to that advised for optic nerve head imaging. The patient should be positioned comfortably on the chin and brow rest. Decrease the distance between the objective and the

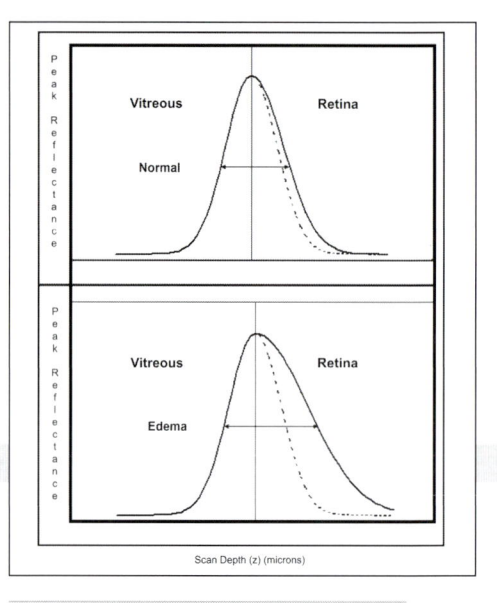

Figure 7.1

In the normal retina, the shape of the confocal intensity profile is slightly asymmetric, with a longer tail toward deeper layers. This is due to light scattered from the deeper retinal tissue, which adds to the high signal of the internal limiting membrane. When edema is present, the amount of scatter from within the edematous retina increases and the peak intensity is reduced. The tail of the confocal intensity profile extends toward the deeper layers, the profile becomes more asymmetric, and its width increases.

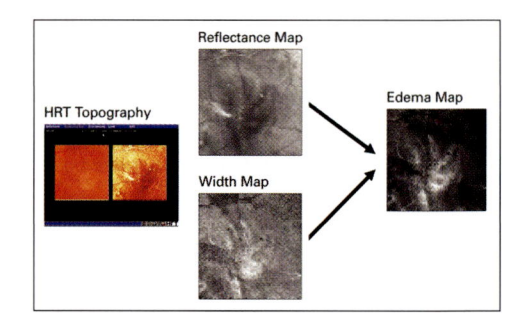

Figure 7.2

The Edema Map is generated by combining information from the Reflectance and Width Maps.

eye until the laser beam appears as a stable, sharp circle on the iris. Then move the laser beam into the center of the pupil. Adjust the camera head position and focus until the brightest, most evenly illuminated image has been found. Recheck the position of the laser beam at the center of the pupil throughout this adjustment period. Focus should be optimized for the retinal vasculature. An external fixation light is required in order to center the retinal area of interest, for example the fovea when screening for diabetic macular edema. If the patient has more than a diopter of astigmatism, it is important to use the HRT astigmatic correction lenses, as the signal width and edema index will otherwise be artifactually increased. Once all these steps have been successfully completed, image acquisition will automatically store three separate image series. If tear film quality is poor, particularly if small circular discontinuities are seen on the video image, use artificial tears to aid image quality. The reflectance topographic standard deviation should be as low as possible and preferably below 30 μm.

IMAGE ANALYSIS

Enter the Heyex Eye Explorer database and select the patient of interest. Once the image icons have appeared in the image window, right-click on the icon and select "Show Movie." If the three image series appear to be well aligned and of similar intensity, then right-click on the icon and select "Compute Retina Map." Figure 7.3 illustrates the window that appears at the end of this process. Select the Reflectance Map and choose one of the four "Contour" options. The cross gives simple crosshairs, with the corresponding profiles being displayed adjacent to the reflectance image (Figure 7.3). The circle gives a default 500-μm-radius circle, corresponding to the Early Treatment of Diabetic Retinopathy Study (ETDRS) criterion for definitions of clinically significant diabetic macular edema.[13,14] If a larger measurement circle is required, select the box at the right side of the circle and drag to the desired radius. The x/y position of the circle and its radius are interactively displayed in millimeters at the bottom right corner of the window. The mean average edema index and signal width for valid pixels within the circle are displayed in the table above. The 9-Zone grid automatically analyzes and tabulates nine regions of the image (Figure 7.4). The center circle has a 500-μm radius. The two larger circles are at 1000 and 1500 μm. As with the circle, the 9-Zone grid can be moved within the image by selecting the box at the center of the display using the left button of the mouse. Note that when positioning the contour a normal fovea will appear as a discrete peak on the reflectance profiles, rather than a pit. This can be a useful anatomic landmark. The final option is a freehand grid that works in a similar way to the contour line drawing utility for the optic nerve. The area of interest can be encapsulated by surrounding with clicks of the left mouse button. This feature is particularly useful when monitoring large, confluent areas of edema, for example as found in branch vein occlusion. Once the contour of choice is appropriately positioned, it can be "Accepted" and the Edema Map selected. Ensure that the Edema Map scale is set to "0 to 4," unless edema index values are extreme. Note that black pixels within the Edema Maps are locations that are considered artifactual. This is due to a variety of reasons including that the signal width could not be modeled (r < 0.85), the pixel was one of the brightest 5%,

Figure 7.3

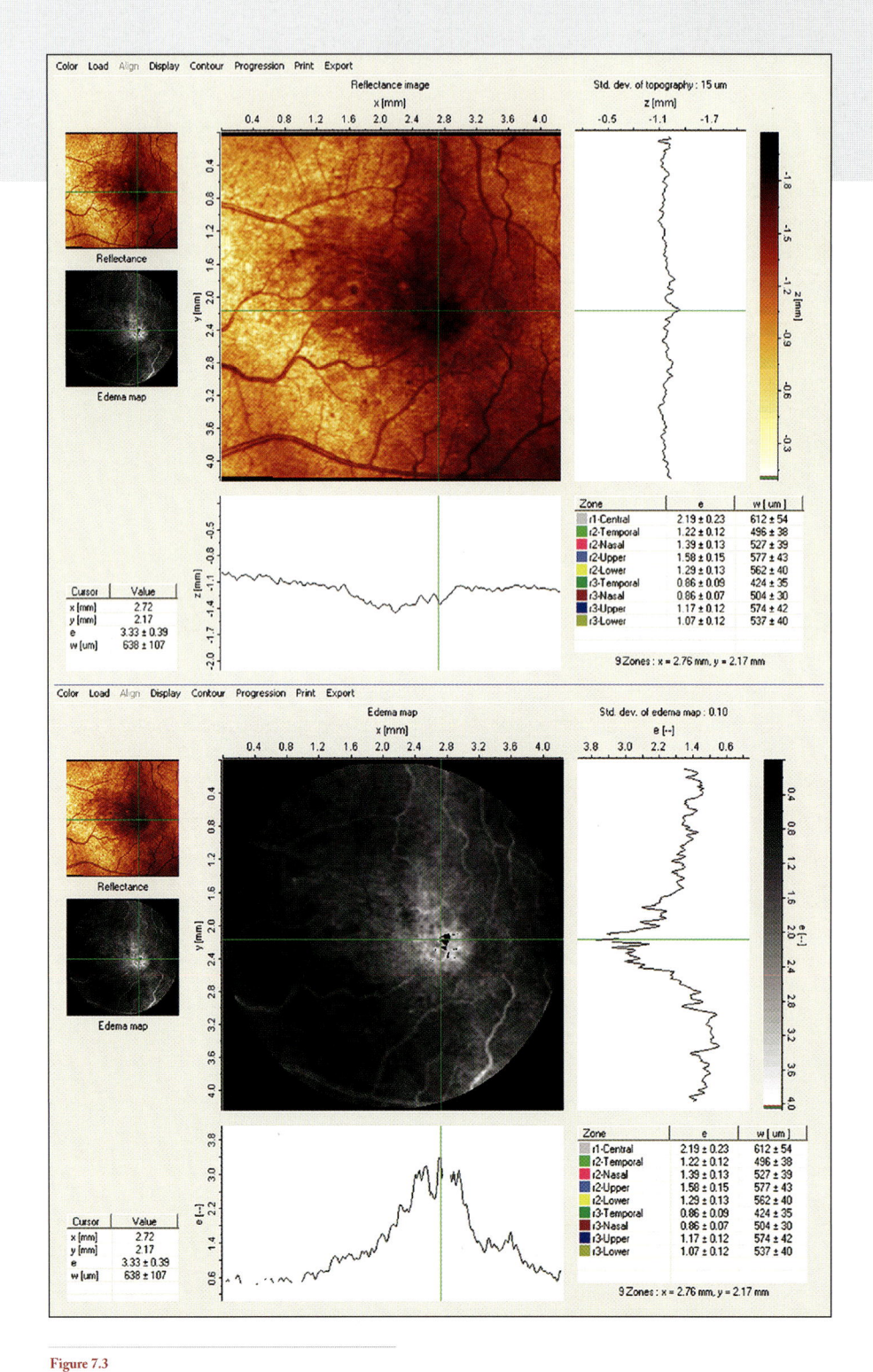

The Retina Module enables the clinician to choose the Reflectance Map or the Edema Map. The crosshairs can be positioned within the image. The profiles are illustrated and associated values are tabulated in the bottom left corner. The case illustrates an example of clinically significant diabetic macular edema.

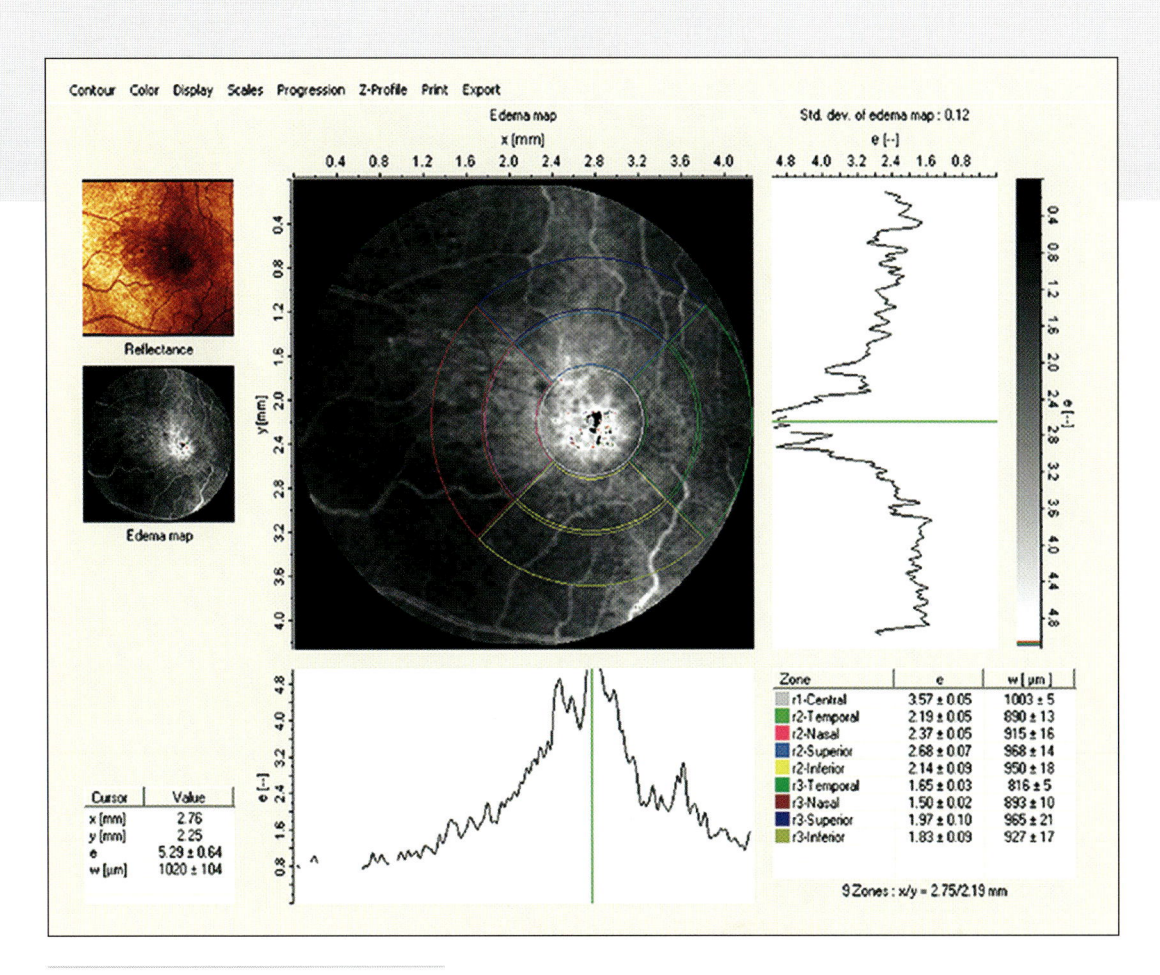

Figure 7.4

The 9-Zone grid is positioned within the Reflectance Map or Edema Map, and values for each area are tabulated in the bottom left corner. The central circle has a diameter of 500 μm. The two larger circles have radii of 1000 and 1500 μm.

and that the pixel was overexposed (gray value > 251). These pixels are labeled as nonvalid and do not influence the edema index calculations. The summary data will be displayed on the printout and can be exported into an Excel® spreadsheet. A table in the bottom left corner of the active window displays the position, edema index, and signal width for the center point of the contour.

Excel is a registered trademark of Microsoft Corporation.

PROGRESSION ANALYSIS

If a retinal condition is being monitored, then the images require alignment to the original baseline image. Unlike the optic nerve module this process is not automatic, due to the diversity and complexity of retinal imaging and the frequent sparsity of anatomical landmarks. To perform the alignment procedure, select the follow-up image in the light box, right-click the mouse, and select "Align." The window that opens will display the baseline and follow-up image and will request that you select four landmarks that are common to both images. It is possible to magnify the image so that locations can be more accurately matched. A number is also displayed that shows the percentage of successful matching in order to assist in optimizing the alignment (100 being the best). It is advisable to use vessel bifurcations and to select a landmark within each quadrant of the images. Once images are aligned and a contour (e.g., the 9-Zone grid) has been positioned on the baseline image, it will be automatically positioned on all subsequent images. A Trend Analysis Graph will be displayed (Figure 7.5).

INTERPRETATION

Normal edema index values for the central 500-µm-radius circle change little with age, and have a value of approximately 1.10 ± 0.30 arbitrary units (au). Normal values are similar for all of the 9-Zone sectors. A value between 1.50 and 1.80 should be considered as borderline and above 1.80 as being outside of normal limits ($p < 0.05$). However, the edema index values are of secondary diagnostic importance to the mapping of discrete areas of increased edema within an image.

It is important to understand that the Edema Maps were developed specifically to map the development of early diabetic edema and its progression. It is assumed that the retina is pigmented, and the edema index will not be calculated reliably in areas of retinal pigment epithelium dropout. The technique can be useful in identifying and monitoring nondiabetic retinal edema, e.g., cystoid macular edema and the edema associated with vein occlusions (Figure 7.6), but will be less useful in macular degeneration. Retinal nevi and prominent macular pigmentation can give artifactually increased edema values, but these are easily identified clinically. In the future it is likely that an estimate of retinal thickness, in micrometers (µm), will be included in the Retina Module as a Thickness Map (Figure 7.7).

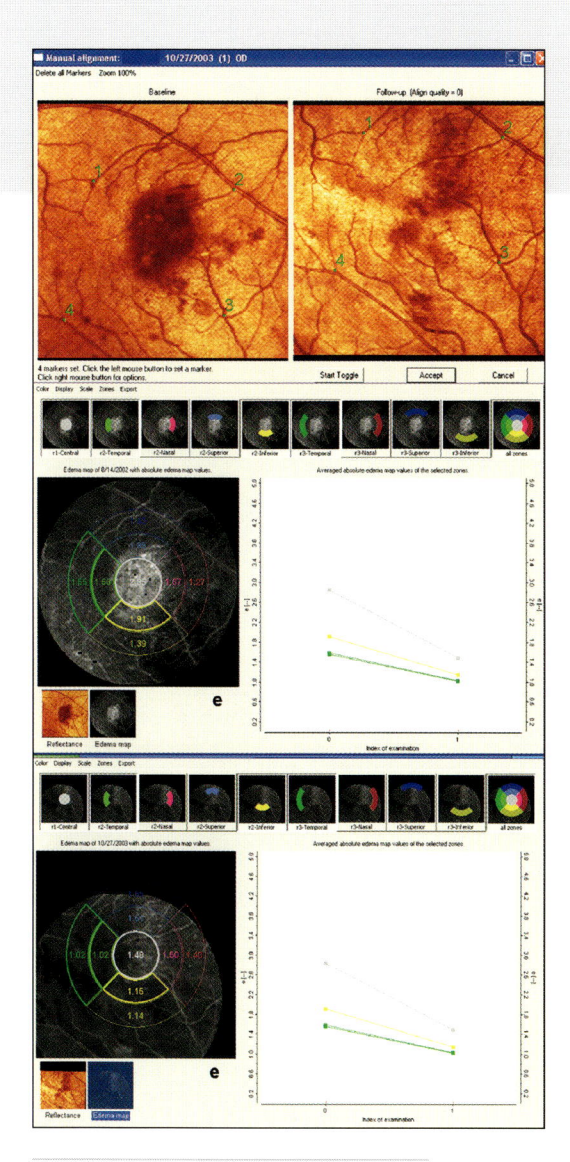

Figure 7.5

Progression Analysis: The upper panel shows the window for the manual alignment utility. Four landmarks are selected that are common to both the baseline image (left) and follow-up image (right). Following alignment the Trend Analysis window will appear after selecting "Progression." The middle panel shows the baseline image for a patient with diabetic macular edema. The lower panel shows a follow-up image taken 14 months later, with a clear reduction in the amount and extent of the edema.

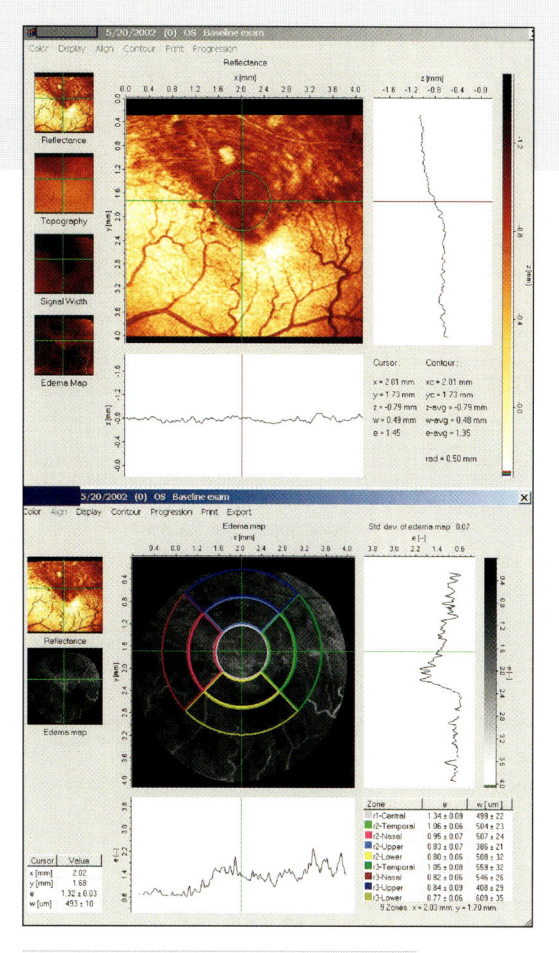

Figure 7.6

Reflectance Map (upper) and Edema Map (lower) showing a case of branch retinal vein occlusion.

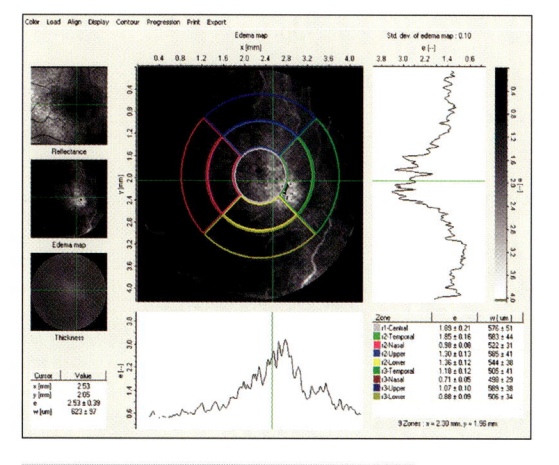

Figure 7.7

Retina Module analysis of a patient with diabetic macular edema (as in Figure 7.4) showing the prototype of the Retinal Thickness Map.

CONCLUSION

In summary, the Retina Module offers a unique and sensitive analysis of the optical effects of edema within the retina. It does so by combining the increase in the signal width experienced as the laser light works its way through the retina, with the reduction in peak reflectance experienced over areas of retinal edema. It does not measure retinal thickness, although retinal edema and retinal thickness are often correlated. The agreement with clinical assessment is good,[9,11] and it is capable of identifying diabetic macular edema prior to its clinical detection.[8,9,11]

REFERENCES

1. Bresnick GH. Diabetic macular edema. *Ophthalmology*. 1986;93:989-997.

2. Bartsch DU, Intaglietta M, Bille JF, Dreher AW, Gharib M, Freeman WR. Confocal laser tomographic analysis of the retina in eyes with macular hole formation and other focal macular diseases. *Am J Ophthalmol*. 1989;108:277-287.

3. Shahidi M, Ogura Y, Blair NP, Zeimer R. Retinal thickness change after focal laser treatment of diabetic macular oedema. *Br J Ophthalmol*. 1994;78:827-830.

4. Puliafito CA, Hee MR, Lin CP, et al. Imaging of macular diseases with optical coherence tomography. *Ophthalmology*. 1995;102:217-229.

5. Hudson C, Charles SJ, Flanagan JG, Brahma AK, Turner GS, McLeod D. Objective morphological assessment of macular hole surgery by scanning laser tomography. *Br J Ophthalmol*. 1997;81:107-116.

6. Hudson C, Flanagan JG, McLeod D, Turner GS. Scanning laser tomography z-profile signal width as an objective index of macular retinal thickening. *Br J Ophthalmol*. 1998;82:121-130.

7. Hudson C, Flanagan JG, Turner GS, Chen H, Young L, McLeod D. Scanning laser-derived edema index topographic maps. In: Wall M, Wild JM, eds. *Perimetry Update 1998/1999*. The Hague: Kugler Publications; 1999:503-510.

8. Hudson C, Flanagan JG, McLeod D. A clinical vision science perspective of the management of diabetic macular oedema. Excerpta Medica. *Focus on Diabetic Retinopathy*. 8:1:4-9.2000.

9. Hudson C, Flanagan JG, Turner GS, Chen HC, Young L, McLeod D. Correlation of a scanning laser derived oedema index and visual function following grid laser treatment for diabetic macular oedema. *Br J Ophthalmol*. 2003;87:455-461.

10. Ferris FL III, Patz A. Macular edema. A complication of diabetic retinopathy. *Surv Ophthalmol*. 1984;28:452-461.

11. Guan K, Hudson C, Flanagan JG. Comparison of the Heidelberg Retina Tomograph II and Retinal Thickness Analyzer in the assessment of diabetic macular edema. *Invest Ophthalmol Vis Sci*. 2004;45:610-616.

12. Eikelboom RH, Cooper RL, Barry CJ. A study of variance in densitometry of retinal nerve fiber layer photographs in normals and glaucoma suspects. *Invest Ophthalmol Vis Sci*. 1990;31:2373-2383.

13. ETDRS Research Group. Early photocoagulation for diabetic retinopathy. ETDRS report number 9. *Ophthalmology*. 1991;98:766-785.

14. Kinyoun J, Barton F, Fisher M, Hubbard L, Aiello L, Ferris F. Detection of diabetic macular edema. Ophthalmoscopy versus photography. ETDRS report number 5. *Ophthalmology*. 1989;96:746-751.

8. Use of the Heidelberg Retina Tomograph (HRT) in the Ocular Hypertension Treatment Study (OHTS)

Linda M. Zangwill, PhD, and Robert N. Weinreb, MD

The Confocal Scanning Laser Ophthalmoscopy (CSLO) Ancillary Study to the Ocular Hypertension Treatment Study (OHTS) was initiated in 1995 to investigate the effectiveness of CSLO (Heidelberg Retina Tomograph [HRT], Heidelberg Engineering, Heidelberg, Germany) to objectively and quantitatively detect glaucomatous changes of the optic disc in ocular hypertensive patients and determine whether CSLO measurements are an accurate predictor of the development of primary open-angle glaucoma (POAG) in ocular hypertensive patients.[1,2] The OHTS, a National Eye Institute–sponsored randomized clinical trial, demonstrated that (1) treatment for ocular hypertension can delay or prevent the onset of POAG; that (2) structural damage is often an early sign of POAG (55% of POAG endpoints were first classified on stereophotograph-based optic disc changes alone); and that (3) baseline stereophotograph-based cup/disc ratio was among the predictors for the onset of POAG.[3-5] With its large cohort of ocular hypertensive participants without clinically evident optic disc or visual field damage at study entry, the OHTS provides a unique opportunity to evaluate whether baseline HRT parameters are associated with the development of POAG in ocular hypertensive patients. This chapter will briefly summarize the CSLO Ancillary Study to the OHTS published cross-sectional results and will describe the results indicating that baseline HRT measurements are significantly associated with the development of POAG.

STUDY DESIGN

Four hundred and fifty-one subjects from seven of the 22 OHTS clinics participated in the CSLO Ancillary Study to the OHTS (Hamilton Glaucoma Center, University of California, San Diego, California; Devers Eye Institute, Portland, Oregon; Henry Ford Medical Center, Troy, Michigan; Jules Stein Eye Institute, University of California, Los Angeles, California; University of California, Davis, California; Scheie Eye Institute, University of Pennsylvania, Philadelphia, Pennsylvania; and New York Eye and Ear Infirmary, New York, New York). All participants met the inclusion and exclusion criteria outlined for the OHTS,[4] that is they had elevated intraocular pressure (IOP) and normal-appearing optic discs and visual fields at study entry. At each CSLO Ancillary Study Center, OHTS participants completed HRT imaging annually at the OHTS dilated visit. Three 10° images centered on the optic disc were obtained on both eyes, and three 15° images were obtained on the right eye. The mean images were used in all analyses. Corneal curvature measurements were used to correct for magnification error, and corrective lenses were used during image acquisition when astigmatism was greater than one diopter. Standardized quality assessment, image processing, and data analysis were completed at the University of California, San Diego CSLO Reading Center.

SUMMARY OF BASELINE CROSS-SECTIONAL RESULTS

The CSLO Ancillary Study to the OHTS baseline publications[1,2] suggested the following:

- HRT stereometric measurements were correlated with stereophotograph-based diameter cup/disc ratio measurements even in OHTS participants with normal-appearing optic discs.[2]

- HRT optic disc measurements describe features that were reflected in standardized assessment of cup/disc diameter ratios from stereophotographs.[2]

- No associations between HRT measurements and gender, diabetes, systemic hypertension, cardiovascular disease, IOP, or visual function were found.[2]

- African Americans had significantly larger mean optic discs, cups, neuroretinal rims, and cup/disc ratios, and smaller mean rim/disc ratios than other OHTS CSLO Ancillary Study participants.[1]

- Racial differences in topographic optic disc parameters could be largely explained by the larger mean optic disc in African American participants compared with other participants.[1]

- Optic disc size should be considered when evaluating the appearance of the optic disc in glaucoma.[1]

DEVELOPMENT OF POAG IN THE OHTS[6]

The primary endpoints for the OHTS were the development of either a confirmed visual field abnormality or a confirmed clinically significant stereophotograph-based optic disc deterioration attributed to POAG. With a median follow-up of 48.4 months for eyes developing POAG, five CSLO Ancillary Study to the OHTS participants developed bilateral POAG and 31 developed unilateral POAG. Of the 41 POAG eyes, nine initially reached endpoint based on visual fields alone, 31 initially on stereophotographs alone, and one based on concurrent visual fields and stereophotographs. The median follow-up of the 432 participants (824 eyes) that did not develop POAG was 84.1 months.

BASELINE HRT MEASUREMENTS ARE ASSOCIATED WITH THE DEVELOPMENT OF POAG[6]

Using the CSLO measurements obtained at entry into the CSLO Ancillary Study to the OHTS, baseline HRT stereometric parameters and indices (HRT classification and Moorfields Regression Analysis [MRA]) were found to be statistically significantly associated with the development of POAG among OHTS participants.[6] (See Table 8.1 adapted from Zangwill et al, *Archives of Ophthalmology*, 2005.[6]) Specifically, compared to a result within normal limits, an overall, global, temporal inferior, and nasal inferior MRA classification as outside normal limits increased the POAG risk by 2.39, 3.37, 5.80, and 4.19, respectively, in multivariate models that controlled for age, IOP, pattern standard deviation, central corneal thickness, history of heart disease, and medication status as a time-dependent covariate. Confidence intervals (CIs) around these estimates were large, with hazards ratios (95% CI) of 2.39, (1.02, 5.62), 3.37 (1.13, 9.99), 5.80 (1.60, 21.00), and 4.19 (1.61, 10.91) respectively. MRA temporal superior region also was associated with the development of POAG, with a hazard ratio (95% CI) of 3.28 (0.98, 10.98).

It should be noted that the majority of eyes with MRA outside normal limits at baseline did not develop POAG within the follow-up period analyzed. The proportion of participants developing POAG with baseline values outside normal limits (positive predictive value) ranged from 14% to 40%. Specifically, among participants with values outside normal limits at baseline, the positive predictive value was 14% by HRT classification (20 of 148), 14% (10 of 71) by MRA overall, 18% (7 of 38) by MRA nasal, 22% (7 of 31) by MRA nasal inferior, 26% (5 of 19) by MRA global, and 40% (4 of 10) by MRA temporal superior. Further analysis is needed to determine whether participants with POAG endpoints and MRA and HRT classification within normal limits at baseline when the visual fields and optic discs photographs were not considered glaucomatous, had measurements outside normal limits during their later follow-up examinations.

On the other hand, the vast majority of eyes with HRT classification or MRA within normal limits did not develop POAG. Specifically, the predictive value of a negative test was high; between 92% and 95% of eyes with HRT classification or MRA within normal limits at baseline did not develop POAG during the follow-up period included in this analysis. These results suggest that HRT indices consistently within normal limits may assist the clinician in identifying ocular hypertensive eyes that have a lower probability of developing glaucoma.

TABLE 8.1: Multivariate Hazard Ratios for the Development of POAG

(Adapted from Zangwill et al, *Archives of Ophthalmology*, 2005 [in press])[6]

		Multivariate* Hazard Ratio (95% CI)
HRT Measures Significantly Associated with the Development of POAG	Mean height contour (per 0.1 mm greater)	2.69 (1.62, 4.49)
	Cup area-to-disc area (per 0.1 greater)	1.25 (1.02, 1.53)
	Mean cup depth (per 0.1 mm greater)	1.60 (1.15, 2.22)
	Reference height (per 0.1 mm greater)	1.49 (1.03, 2.17)
	Rim area (per 0.2 greater)	0.57 (0.42, 0.78)
	Rim area/disc area (per 0.1 greater)	0.76 (0.62, 0.93)
	Rim volume above reference (per 0.1 mm³ greater)	0.65 (0.47, 0.91)
HRT Measures Not Significantly Associated with the Development of POAG	Disc area (per 0.4 mm² greater)	0.86 (0.57, 1.30)
	Cup area (per 0.3 mm² greater)	1.21 (0.96, 1.53)
	RNFL thickness (per 0.1 mm greater)	0.66 (0.35, 1.23)
	Cup shape (per 0.1 greater)	1.02 (0.62, 1.67)
	Cup volume below surface (per 0.1 mm³ greater)	1.10 (0.97, 1.25)
	RNFL cross-sectional area (per 0.3 mm³ greater)	0.72 (0.48, 1.06)
	Cup volume below reference (per 0.1 mm³ greater)	1.20 (1.01, 1.43)
HRT Indices Associated with the Development of POAG (outside normal limits versus not)	HRT classification	2.54 (1.31, 4.90)
	MRA overall	2.39 (1.02, 5.62)
	MRA global	3.37 (1.13, 9.99)
	MRA temporal inferior	5.80 (1.60, 21.00)
	MRA temporal superior	3.28 (0.98, 10.98)
	MRA nasal inferior	4.19 (1.61, 10.91)
HRT Indices Not Associated with the Development of POAG (outside normal limits versus not)	MRA nasal superior	0.72 (0.11, 4.63)
	MRA nasal	1.59 (0.48, 5.24)
	MRA temporal	2.48 (0.66, 9.22)

* Multivariate model contains baseline age, intraocular pressure, pattern standard deviation, central corneal thickness, and history of heart disease, with medication status as a time-dependent covariate; 112 eyes were excluded from the multivariate analyses due to missing central corneal thickness values.

In addition to the HRT indices, stereometric parameters also were significantly associated with the development of POAG in participants of the CSLO Ancillary Study to the OHTS. A larger baseline HRT mean height contour, mean cup depth, cup area-to-disc area, and cup volume below reference, and a smaller rim area, rim volume, and rim area-to-disc area were significantly associated with the development of POAG in multivariate models. These results are similar to the OHTS finding that a larger baseline stereophotograph-based vertical cup/disc ratio was predictive of the onset of POAG with a multivariate hazards ratio (per .1 larger) of 1.32 (1.19–1.47).[3] As our cross-sectional analysis found that the larger optic cups, neuroretinal rims, and cup/disc ratios in African Americans compared with other participants could be explained by their larger disc size, we hypothesized that a large disc may be a significant predictor of the development of POAG in OHTS participants. The results of the current analysis did not confirm this hypothesis; disc area was not significantly associated with the development of POAG.

It should be noted that due to the limited number of POAG endpoints, stereophotograph-based cup/disc ratios were not included in the multivariate models at this time, as the measurements are highly correlated with HRT parameters. Therefore, this study did not yet determine whether the OHTS prediction model that includes baseline HRT measurements is improved over one that includes baseline stereophotograph cup/disc ratio measurements. This analysis will be completed in the future, when a larger number of POAG endpoints are available to adequately address this issue.

Although several HRT measurements were consistent predictors of POAG in the multivariate models, the large confidence intervals with the proximity of the lower confidence limit to one and the limited positive predictive value of the indices suggest that it is not prudent to rely on a single parameter when making clinical decisions. Longer follow-up is needed to better estimate the true predictive ability of the HRT measures. Moreover, as highlighted in other chapters of this primer, clinical decisions should be based on using HRT results with other clinical tools including the clinical examination and tests of visual function.

RESULTS OF BASELINE HRT ASSOCIATIONS WITH THE DEVELOPMENT OF POAG

- Baseline HRT stereometric optic disc parameters and HRT indices are significantly associated with the development of POAG in OHTS participants.

- The vast majority of eyes (92% to 95%) with an MRA result within normal limits at baseline did not develop POAG during the follow-up period.

- Further analysis is needed to determine whether participants with POAG endpoints and baseline HRT results within normal limits (when their visual fields and optic discs also did not appear glaucomatous) had measurements outside normal limits during their later follow-up examinations.

REFERENCES

1. Zangwill LM, Weinreb RN, Berry CC, et al. Racial differences in optic disc topography: baseline results from the confocal scanning laser ophthalmoscopy ancillary study to the ocular hypertension treatment study. *Arch Ophthalmol.* 2004;122:22-28.

2. Zangwill LM, Weinreb RN, Berry CC, et al. The confocal scanning laser ophthalmoscopy ancillary study to the ocular hypertension treatment study: study design and baseline factors. *Am J Ophthalmol.* 2004;137:219-227.

3. Gordon MO, Beiser JA, Brandt JD, et al. The Ocular Hypertension Treatment Study: baseline factors that predict the onset of primary open-angle glaucoma. *Arch Ophthalmol.* 2002;120:714-720.

4. Gordon MO, Kass MA. The Ocular Hypertension Treatment Study: design and baseline description of the participants. *Arch Ophthalmol.* 1999;117:573-583.

5. Kass MA, Heuer DK, Higginbotham EJ, et al. The Ocular Hypertension Treatment Study: a randomized trial determines that topical ocular hypotensive medication delays or prevents the onset of primary open-angle glaucoma. *Arch Ophthalmol.* 2002;120:701-713.

6. Zangwill LM, Weinreb RN, Beiser JA, et al. Baseline topographic optic disc measurements are associated with the development of primary open angle glaucoma: the Confocal Scanning Laser Ophthalmoscopy Ancillary Study to the Ocular Hypertension Treatment Study. *Arch Ophthalmol.* 2005 (in press).

9 The Importance of Optic Nerve Imaging in Clinical Practice

Jeffrey M. Liebmann, MD

Glaucoma is a disease of the optic nerve characterized by a specific pattern of progressive injury to retinal ganglion cells and their axons, which results in alteration of optic disc topography, commonly known as "cupping," and associated visual field loss. Glaucoma is, therefore, a disease that is defined, staged, longitudinally assessed, and treated based upon the structural appearance of the optic nerve and its function. While intraocular pressure reduction remains the mainstay of therapy, assessment for progressive disease depends solely on periodic assessment of the structure and function of the optic nerve. Careful, accurate assessment and documentation of the appearance of the optic disc become indispensable for diagnosis and disease management. Perhaps more importantly, documentation of the appearance of the optic disc is critical to longitudinal patient care.

Clinical evaluation of the optic disc is based upon assessment of the optic nerve during the ophthalmic examination. In the past, this was performed with direct ophthalmoscopy or slit-lamp biomicroscopy with the aid of a Hruby lens. In current practice, clinical stereoscopic examination of the optic disc at the slit-lamp is achieved with a handheld indirect lens (60, 78, or 90 diopter) and indirect ophthalmoscopy. Each of these techniques has its own advantages and disadvantages, but all purely clinical approaches to optic disc evaluation are limited by their subjective nature.

Documentation of the appearance of the optic disc at baseline is most often achieved with standard stereophotography. Clinical examination and review of stereophotographs provide a method for qualitative assessment of the optic disc, but provide only limited quantitative information. The recognition of the intrinsic relationship between the optic nerve and disease management and the need for a more quantitative approach to optic nerve assessment has been an underlying driving force for the development of confocal scanning laser ophthalmoscopy.

Confocal scanning laser ophthalmoscopy of the optic disc using the Heidelberg Retina Tomograph II (HRT II) provides detailed, precise, quantitative information about the contour of the optic disc that is invaluable in the assessment of the optic disc and has altered our approach to the optic disc examination. Clinicians are now able to quantify the amount of neuroretinal rim and describe its features in great detail. In addition to global assessment of rim area, measurable features of the optic disc now include focal loss of neural rim, volumetric assessment of the rim and cup, precise assessment of disc area, evaluation of the shape of the cup, and characteristics of the retinal nerve fiber layer, among others.

This quantitative information allows for easier detection of disease by identifying features of the disc that are more typical of glaucoma than normal individuals. Computer-assisted analysis, such as the information revealed by Moorfields Regression Analysis, aids the clinician in initial diagnosis by revealing structural features and relationships of the optic disc that are both not evident during clinical examination and require computerized interpretation of large amounts of data.

Although the wide biologic variability in the appearance of the normal optic disc makes the diagnosis of glaucoma difficult in some patients even with the aid of quantitative information, longitudinal assessment of quantitative information can provide earlier determination of disease progression. This aids not only in the assessment of established disease, but also assists in the initial diagnosis of the disease by detecting subtle changes in optic disc topography that are not visible by clinical examination or more traditional methods of optic nerve assessment. These early quantifiable changes in disc topography most often precede any reliable, detectable changes in traditional, achromatic perimetric measures of visual function. One of the key purposes of this book is to help clinicians translate these scientific advances into clinical practice and the care of patients.

This revolution in our approach to optic disc imaging parallels the introduction of automated perimetry. Early versions of the automated perimeter were limited by available hardware and software, lack of good normative databases, and lack of clinical experience. Although it took many years for automated perimetry to gain widespread acceptance, this technology is now the gold standard for evaluation of visual function. The same process of instrument development applies to the HRT, which in the HRT II combines high technology, ease of use, a normative database, and algorithms to aid in the differentiation of normal from abnormal and detection of progression. The information gleaned from automated optic nerve assessment is more reliable and reproducible and will likely be more sensitive and specific than subjective interpretation of disc photographs for most practitioners.

Where is our new technology leading? The integration of new scientific information into clinical practice is often difficult for the busy clinician. Information provided by the HRT II improves patient care by augmenting clinical assessment of the optic nerve, allowing us to move beyond subjective interpretation of the optic nerve to data-driven decision-making. New evidence from longitudinal studies involving HRT assessment of optic disc parameters will serve to enhance our understanding not only of glaucoma pathophysiology, risk assessment, and the relationship between structural and functional alteration in glaucoma, but also will enable us to more appropriately initiate therapy and advance therapy when indicated. This process of a more directed therapeutic approach offers us the opportunity to fine-tune our therapy by minimizing it in persons with only modest amounts of nerve injury, while maximizing it in those that are progressing toward blindness. Given the need for accurate disc assessment, it is highly likely that each of us will have an imaging device as part of our routine ophthalmic practice and that it will play an integral role in the management of persons with glaucoma and those at risk for this blinding disease.

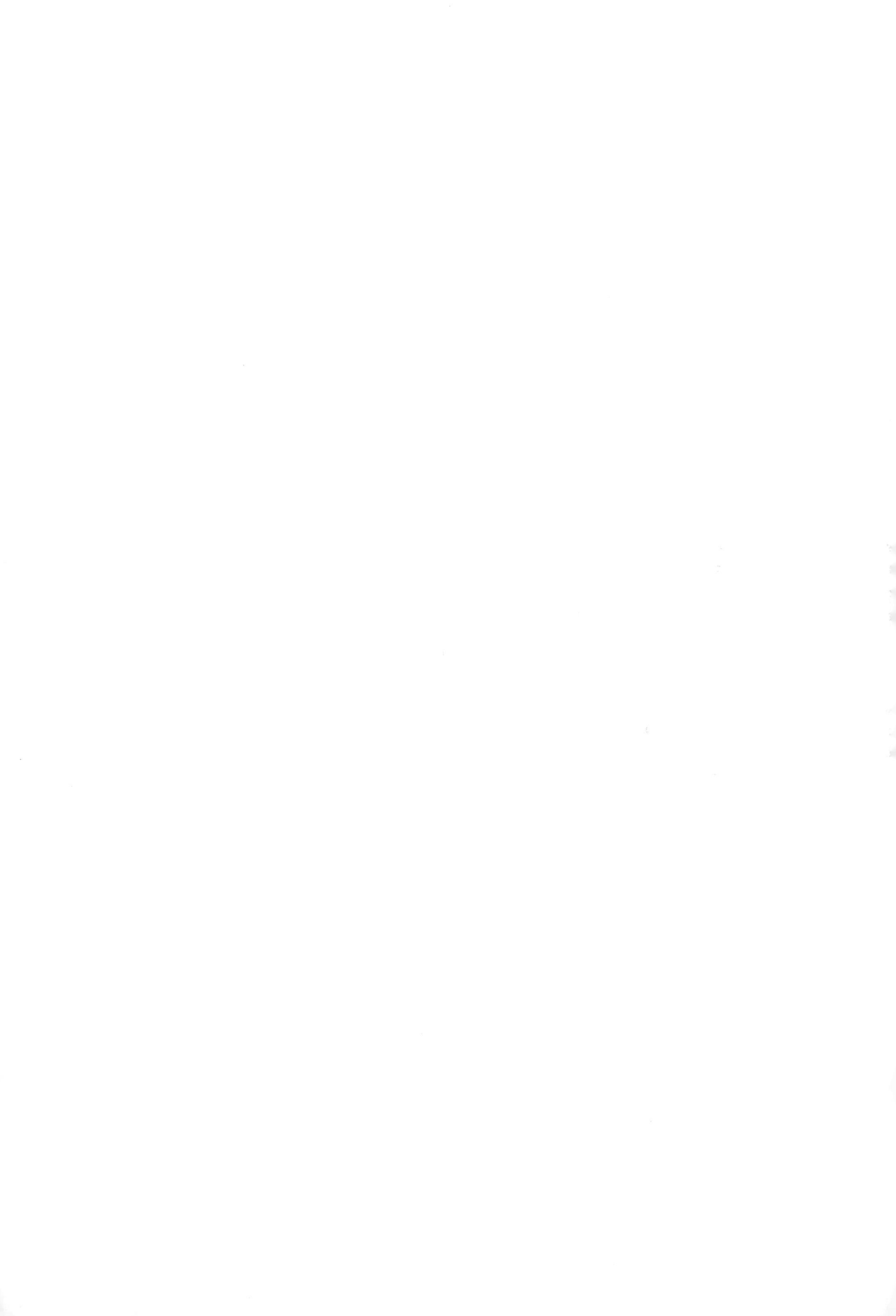

HRT II PRIMER CASES
Murray Fingeret, OD

GLAUCOMA DIAGNOSIS

1. An individual with primary open-angle glaucoma is seen with optic nerve damage worse in the left eye. Moorfields analysis shows several sectors to be flagged for OD, and the temporal inferior (TI) height around the contour line is depressed. The disc is 2.3 mm^2 in area, with the rim area, rim volume, cup shape measure, and mean RNFL thickness below the normative range. The disc area for OS is 2.126 mm^2, and the rim area, rim volume, cup shape measure, height variation contour, and mean RNFL are all flagged as being outside the normal limits. Three sectors inferiorly are flagged on Moorfields analysis, with a reduced RNFL height visible inferiorly on the height around the contour line. For the OU printout, the OS contour line is reduced as compared to OD. Both images are excellent quality (Standard deviation 10 μm OD, 9 μm). This individual has glaucomatous damage, worse both inferiorly as well as greater in the OS.

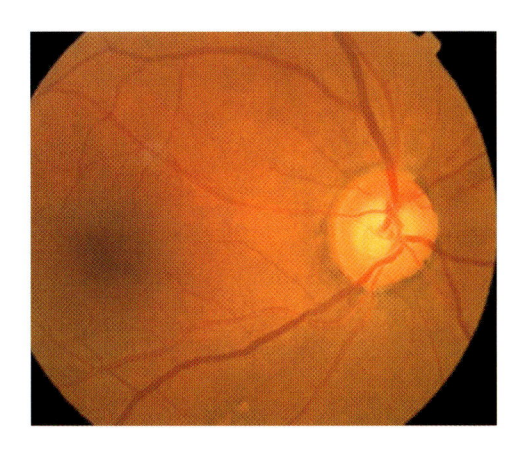

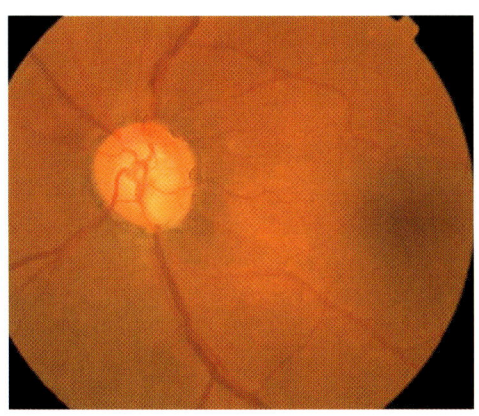

96 FINGERET | HRT II Primer Cases

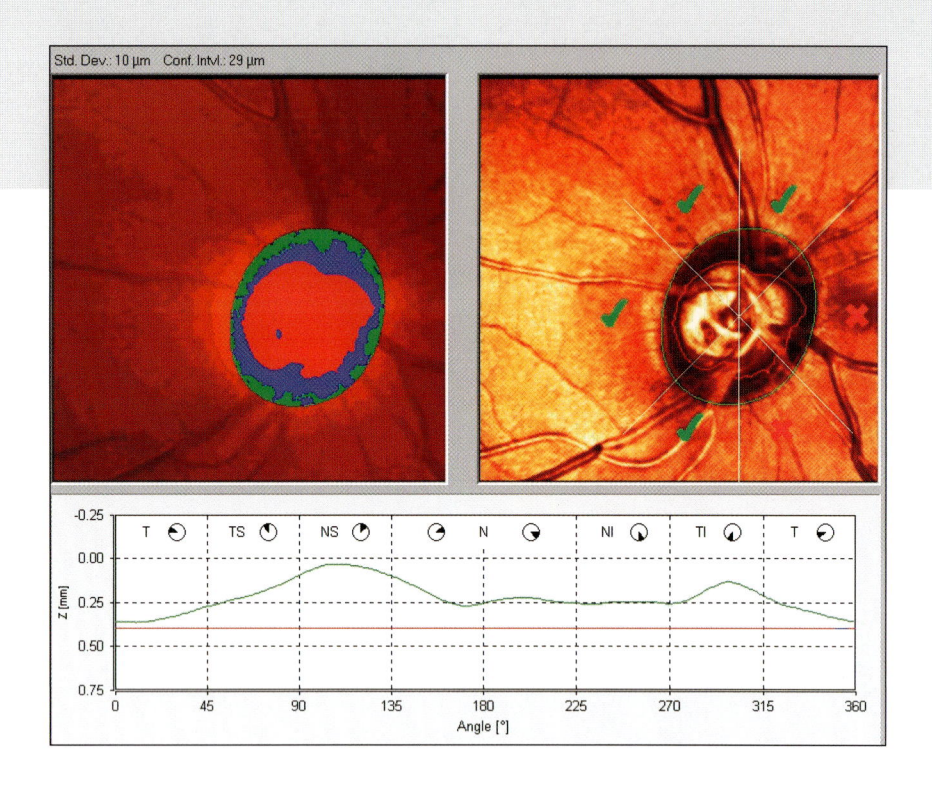

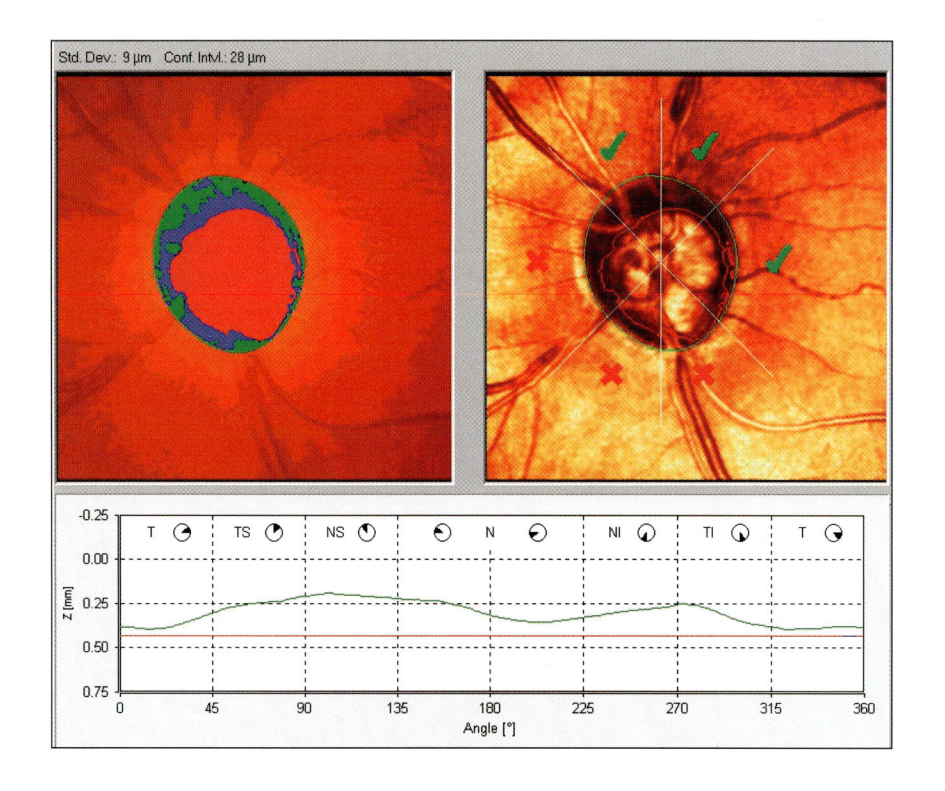

Heidelberg Retina Tomograph II
OU Quickview

Patient:
Sex: male DOB: 1933 Pat-ID: ---

Examination: Date: Sep/25/2003

OD
Focus: 3.00 dpt Depth: 2.50 mm Operator: --- IOP: ---
Std Dev: 10 µm

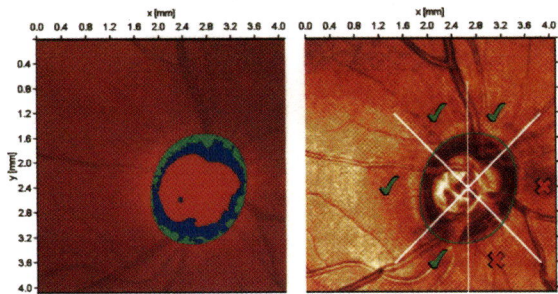

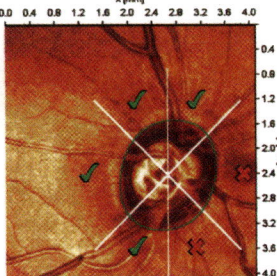

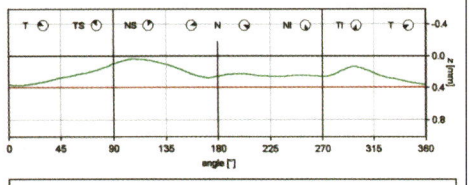

Stereometric Analysis		Normal
Rim Area	1.152 mm²	1.20 - 1.78
Rim Volume	0.182 cmm	0.24 - 0.49
Linear Cup/Disk Ratio	0.709	0.36 - 0.80
Cup Shape Measure	-0.111	-0.27 - -0.09
Height Variation Contour	0.332 mm	0.30 - 0.47
Mean RNFL Thickness	0.177 mm	0.18 - 0.31

OS
Focus: 3.00 dpt Depth: 3.25 mm Operator: --- IOP: ---
Std Dev: 9 µm

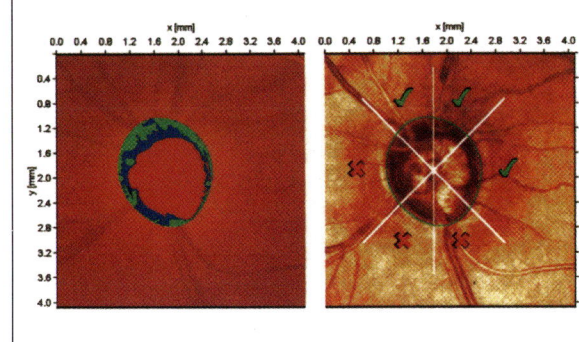

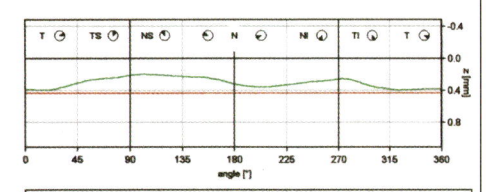

Stereometric Analysis		Normal
Rim Area	0.851 mm²	1.20 - 1.78
Rim Volume	0.122 cmm	0.24 - 0.49
Linear Cup/Disk Ratio	0.774	0.36 - 0.80
Cup Shape Measure	-0.020	-0.27 - -0.09
Height Variation Contour	0.204 mm	0.30 - 0.47
Mean RNFL Thickness	0.130 mm	0.18 - 0.31

OU - Current Exam
- OD contour line
- OS contour line

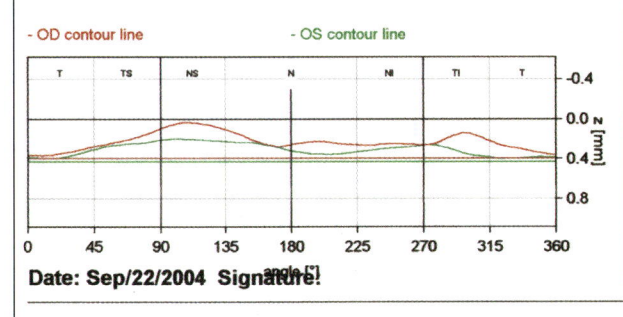

Date: Sep/22/2004 Signature!

Comments:

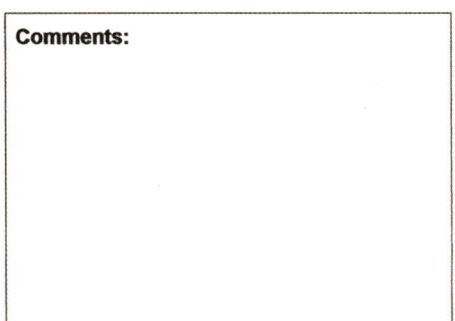

Software: IR1-V1.7/900

2. HRT II images are seen for an individual diagnosed as a glaucoma suspect due to large cupping. The intraocular pressure was in the low teens, corneal thickness 550 μm in each eye, and the Humphrey 24-2 SITA Standard visual fields were full in each eye. The disc area was 4.06 mm^2 OD and 4.71 mm^2 OS, which is indicative of very large optic nerve heads. While several sectors are flagged on Moorfields analysis, this is often seen in eyes in which the optic nerves are very large. The height around the contour line appears adequate and most of the stereometric parameters are within normal limits. This is an individual with physiologic cupping associated with a large optic disc.

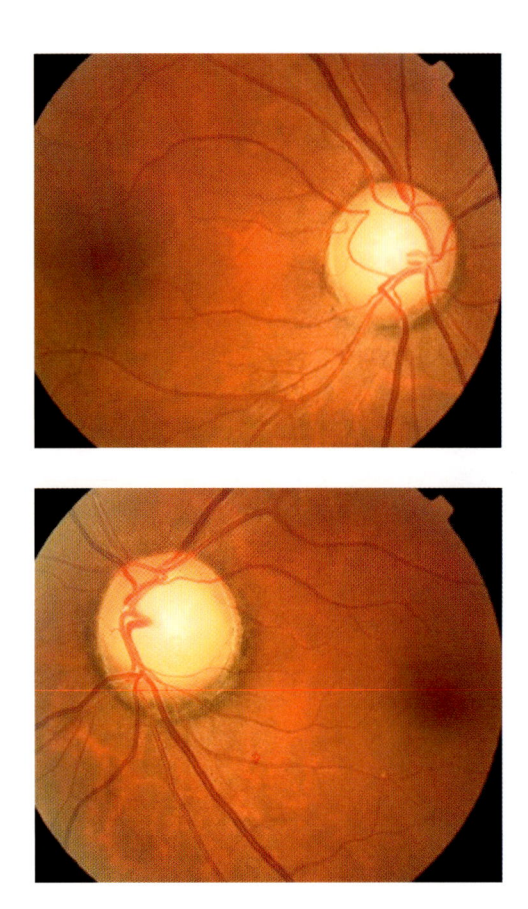

HRT II Primer Cases | FINGERET 99

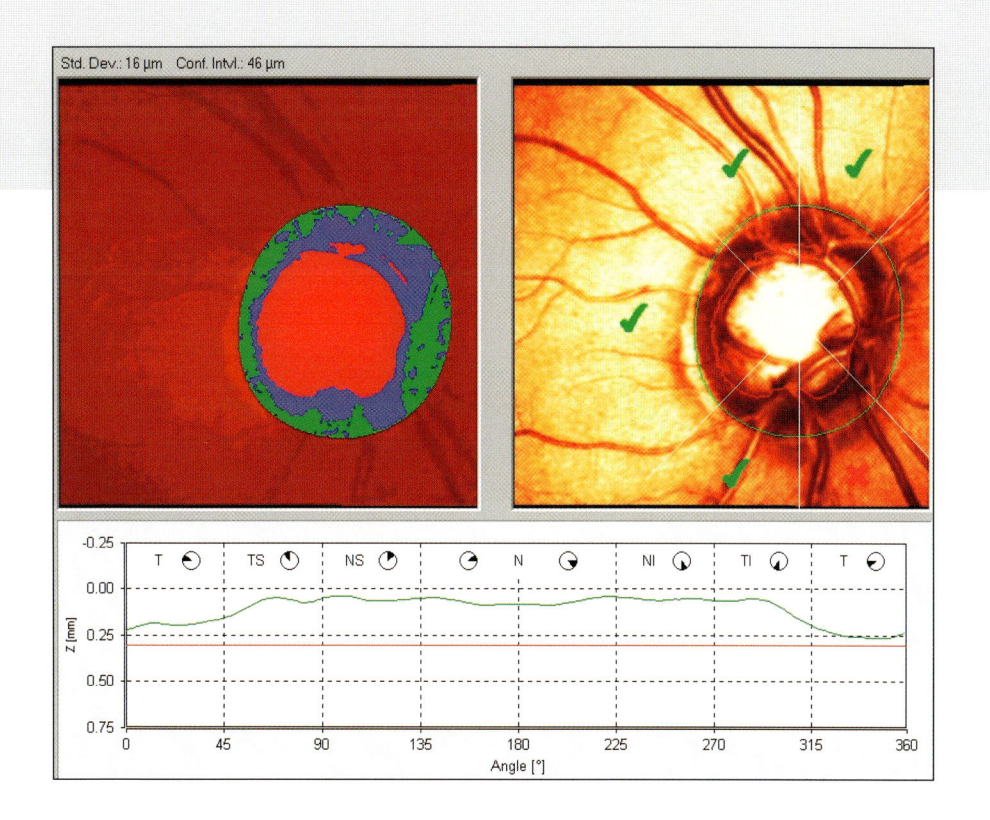

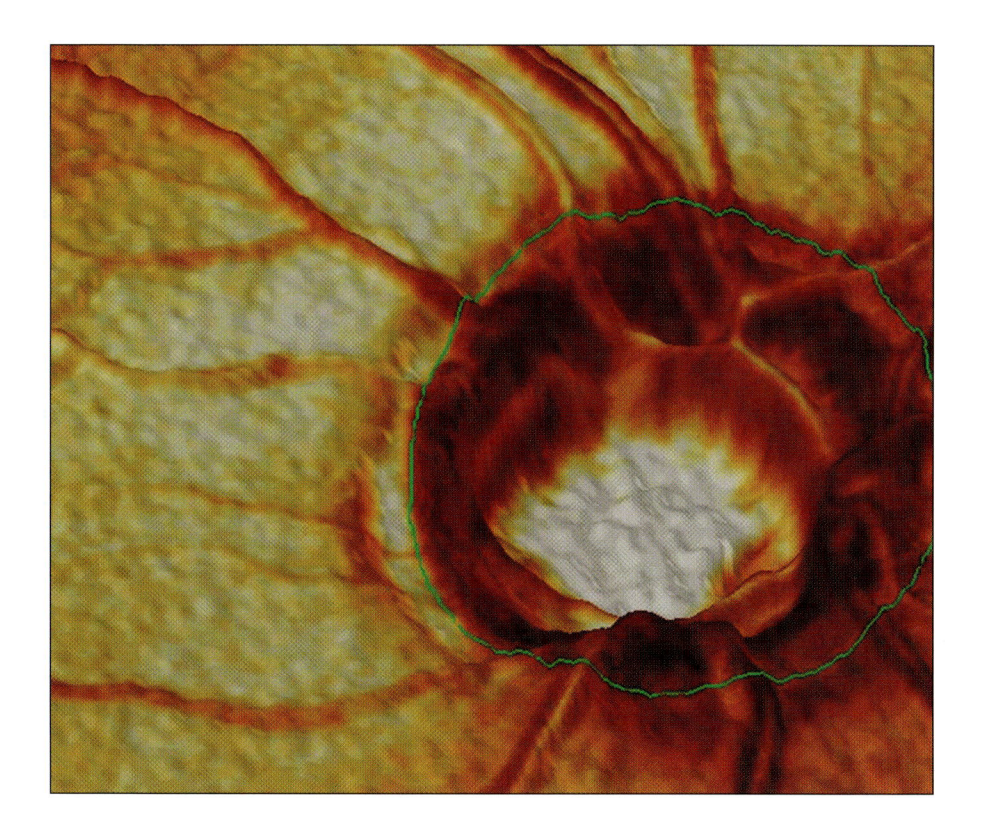

100 FINGERET | HRT II Primer Cases

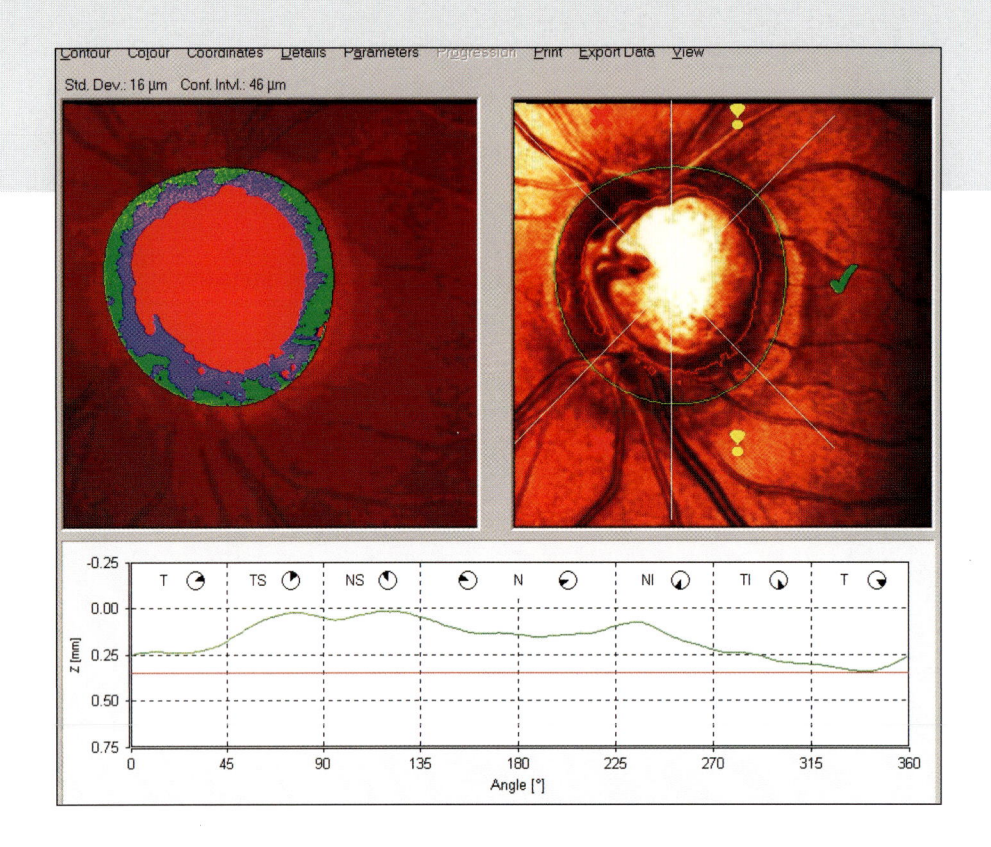

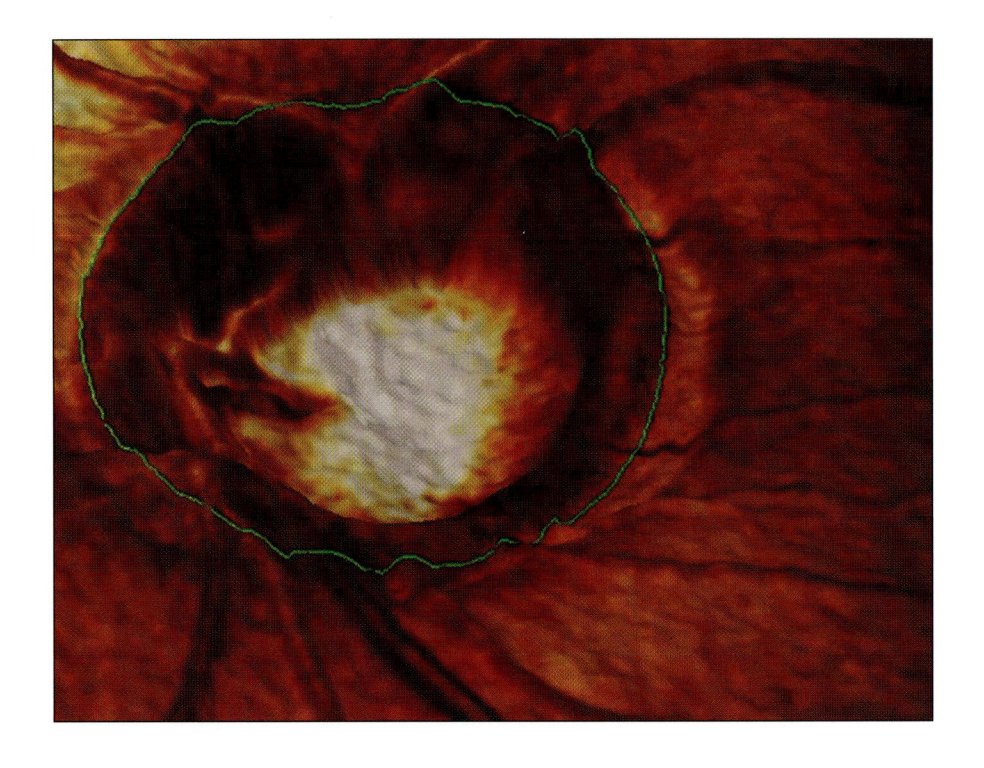

Heidelberg Retina Tomograph II
OU Quickview

Patient: Sex: male DOB: 1953 Pat-ID: ---

Examination: Date: Apr/10/2003

OD
Focus: 1.00 dpt Depth: 3.75 mm Operator: --- IOP: ---
Std Dev: 16 µm

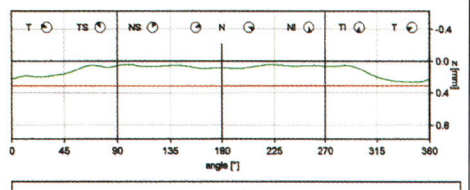

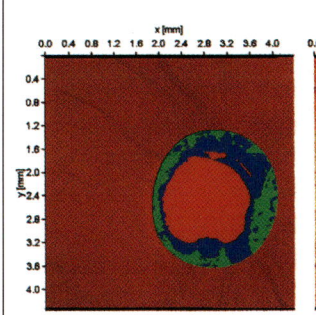

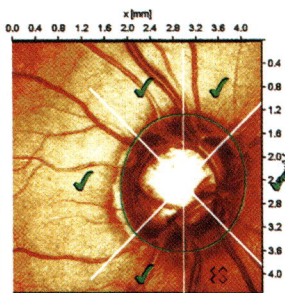

Stereometric Analysis		Normal
Rim Area	2.260 mm²	1.20 - 1.78
Rim Volume	0.413 cmm	0.24 - 0.49
Linear Cup/Disk Ratio	0.666	0.36 - 0.80
Cup Shape Measure	-0.104	-0.27 - -0.09
Height Variation Contour	0.225	0.30 - 0.47
Mean RNFL Thickness	0.201 mm	0.18 - 0.31

OS
Focus: 1.00 dpt Depth: 3.00 mm Operator: --- IOP: ---
Std Dev: 16 µm

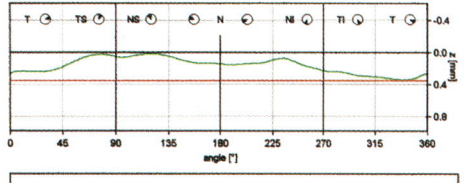

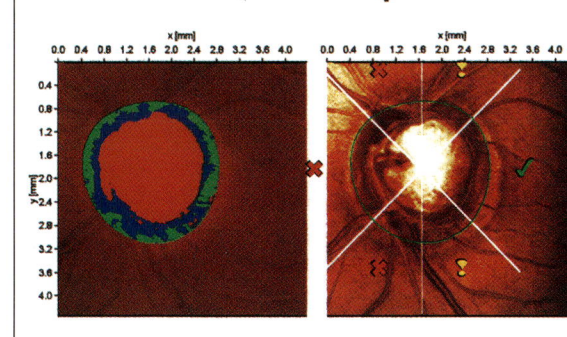

Stereometric Analysis		Normal
Rim Area	2.034 mm²	1.20 - 1.78
Rim Volume	0.309 cmm	0.24 - 0.49
Linear Cup/Disk Ratio	0.754	0.36 - 0.80
Cup Shape Measure	-0.009	-0.27 - -0.09
Height Variation Contour	0.327	0.30 - 0.47
Mean RNFL Thickness	0.185 mm	0.18 - 0.31

OU - Current Exam
- OD contour line
- OS contour line

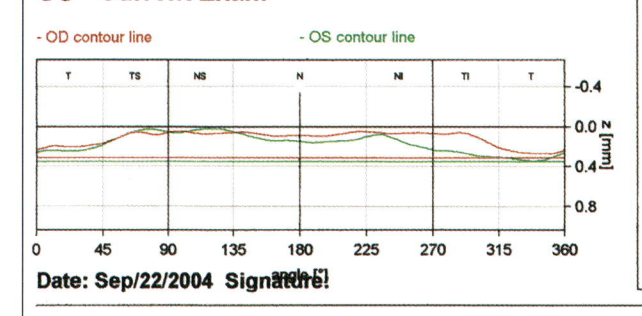

Comments:

Date: Sep/22/2004 Signature!

Software: IR1-V1.7/900

3. This individual was diagnosed as a glaucoma suspect, based upon cup/disc ratio asymmetry. The HRT II printout shows the cup/disc asymmetry to be due to optic nerve size asymmetry. The right nerve is larger (2.2 mm^2), while the left eye is 1.18 mm^2.

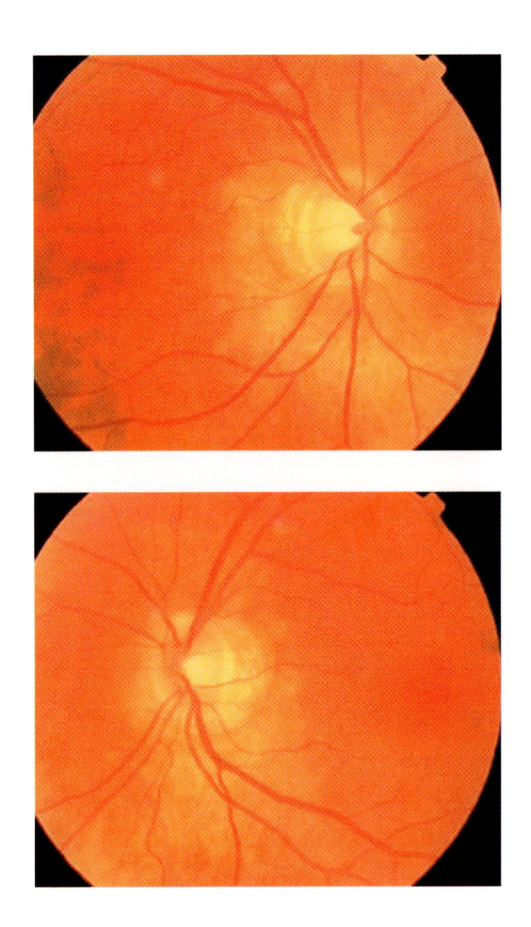

HRT II Primer Cases | FINGERET 103

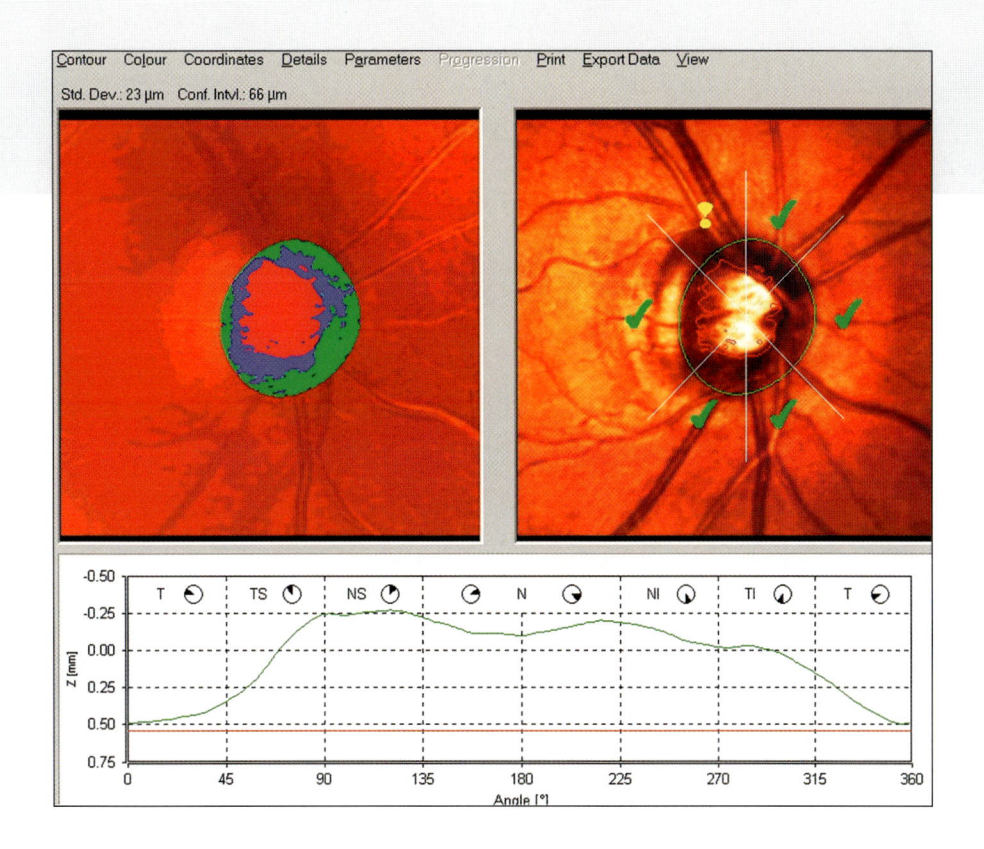

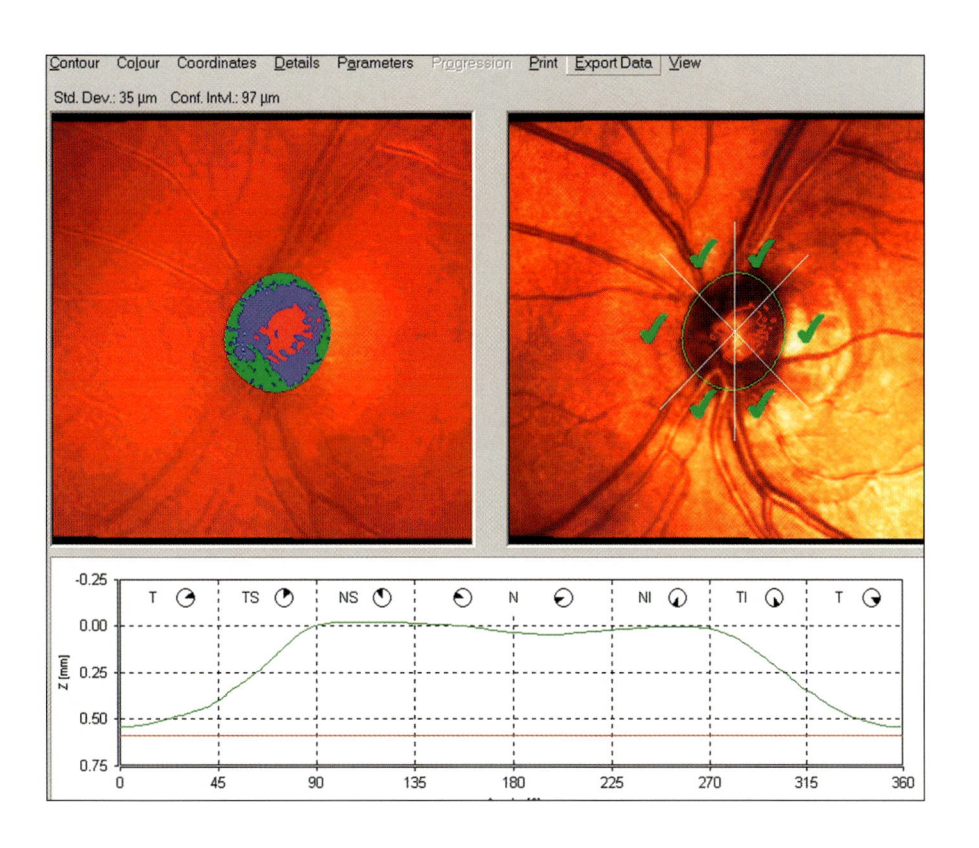

Heidelberg Retina Tomograph II
OU Quickview

HEIDELBERG ENGINEERING

Patient: Sex: male   DOB: 1946   Pat-ID: ---

Examination: Date: Apr/2/2002

OD
Focus: -9.00 dpt   Depth: 3.75 mm   Operator: ---   IOP: ---

Std Dev: 23 µm

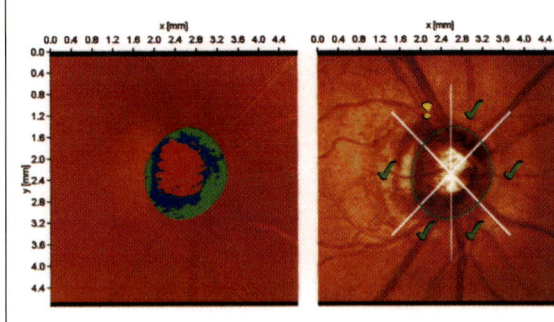

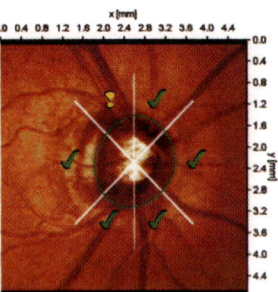

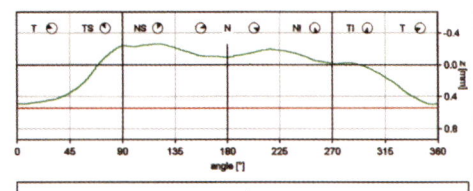

Stereometric Analysis		Normal
Rim Area	1.400 mm²	1.20 - 1.78
Rim Volume	0.699 cmm	0.24 - 0.49
Linear Cup/Disk Ratio	0.603	0.36 - 0.80
Cup Shape Measure	-0.118	-0.27 - -0.09
Height Variation Contour	0.763 mm	0.30 - 0.47
Mean RNFL Thickness	0.514 mm	0.18 - 0.31

OS
Focus: -5.00 dpt   Depth: 2.75 mm   Operator: ---   IOP: ---

Std Dev: 35 µm

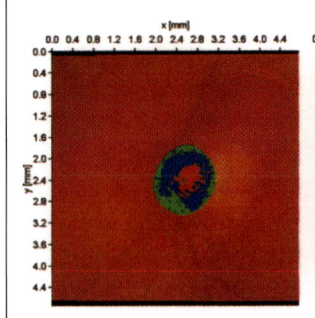

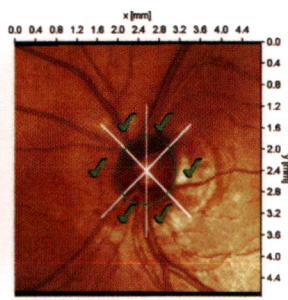

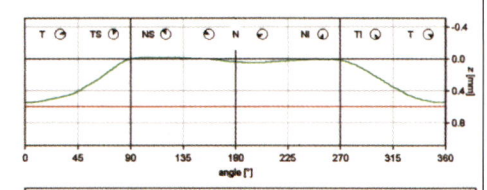

Stereometric Analysis		Normal
Rim Area	0.977 mm²	1.20 - 1.78
Rim Volume	0.348 cmm	0.24 - 0.49
Linear Cup/Disk Ratio	0.421	0.36 - 0.80
Cup Shape Measure	-0.160	-0.27 - -0.09
Height Variation Contour	0.563 mm	0.30 - 0.47
Mean RNFL Thickness	0.421 mm	0.18 - 0.31

OU - Current Exam
- OD contour line   - OS contour line

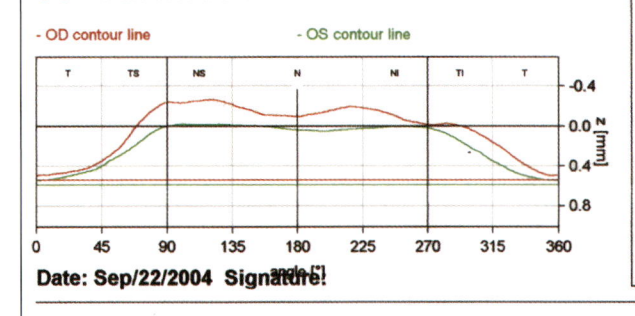

Comments:

Date: Sep/22/2004   Signature:

Software: IR1-V1.7/900

4. This individual has primary open-angle glaucoma, worse in the left eye. Nerve fiber layer dropout is seen in both eyes, but larger and in a wedge shape OS. The HRT II printout shows several sectors flagged in each eye with Moorfields analysis. The rim area, rim volume, cup shape measure, and height variation contour is below normal limits in both eyes, with the mean RNFL reduced in OS only. The large cup is visible as seen as red on the topography image, while the rim area is thin (blue and green). The images are of excellent quality, as both have low standard deviations.

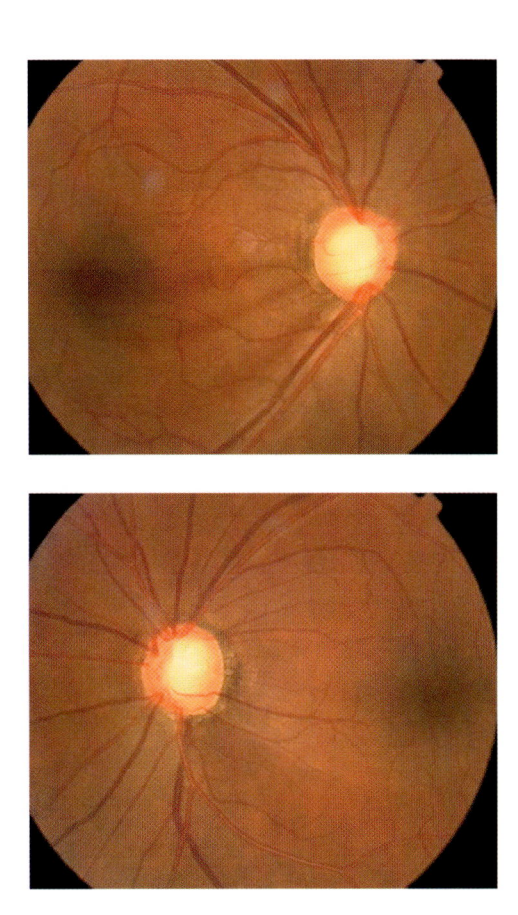

106 FINGERET | HRT II Primer Cases

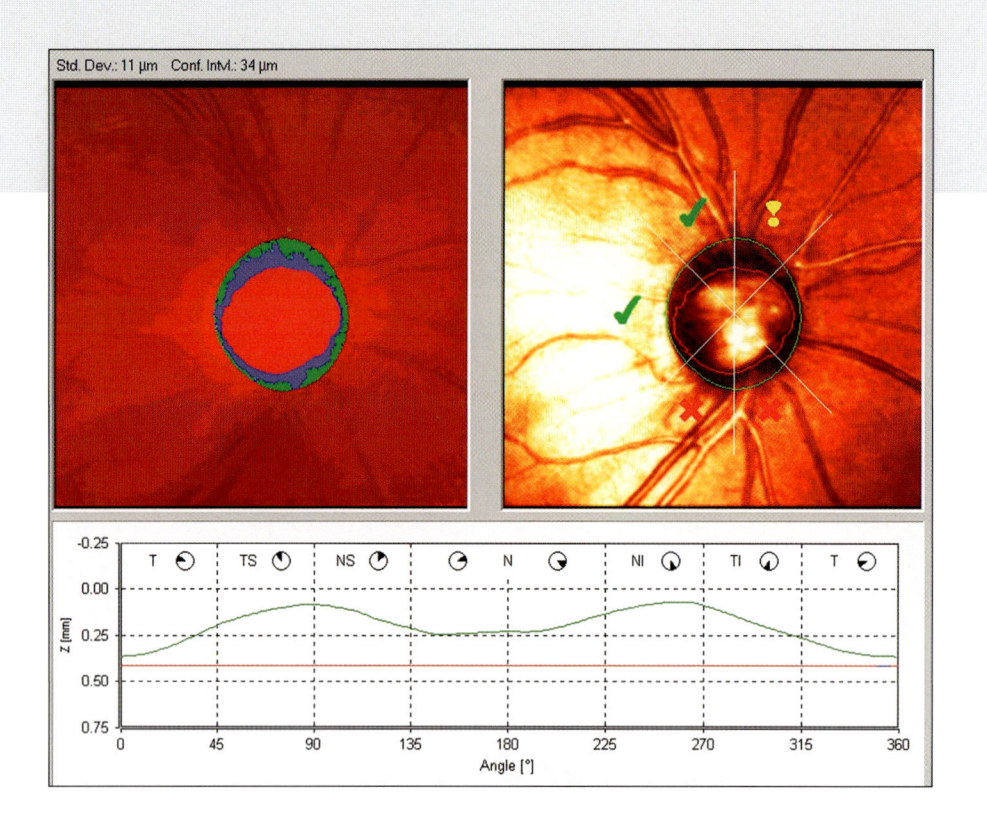

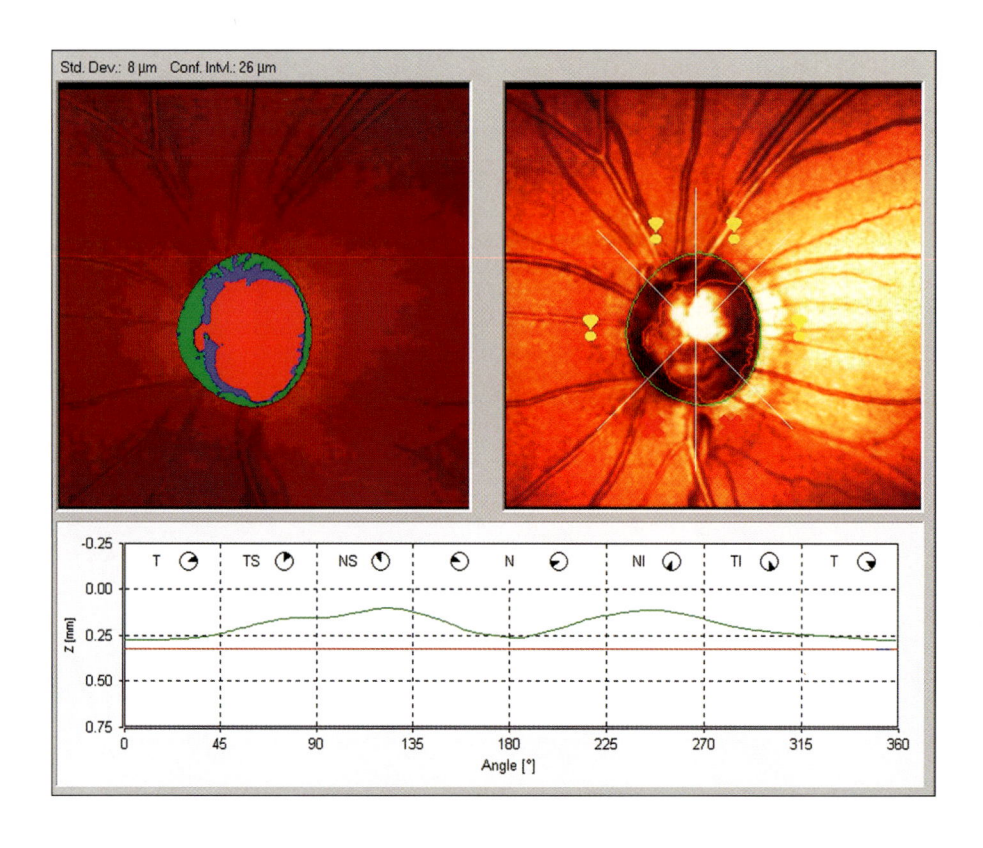

Heidelberg Retina Tomograph II
OU Quickview

Patient: Sex: male DOB: 1951 Pat-ID: 9863

Examination: Date: Nov/17/2003

OD
Focus: -2.00 dpt Depth: 3.00 mm Operator: --- IOP: ---
Std Dev: 11 µm

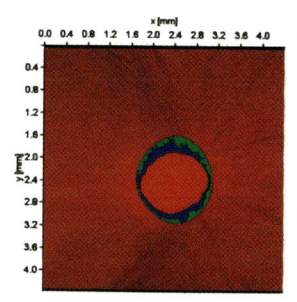

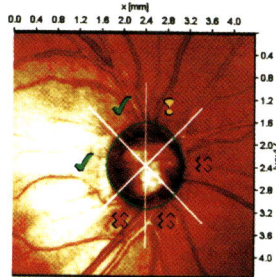

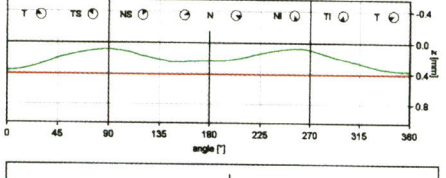

Stereometric Analysis		Normal
Rim Area	0.672 mm²	1.20 - 1.78
Rim Volume	0.139 cmm	0.24 - 0.49
Linear Cup/Disk Ratio	0.780	0.36 - 0.80
Cup Shape Measure	-0.004	-0.27 - -0.09
Height Variation Contour	0.296 mm	0.30 - 0.47
Mean RNFL Thickness	0.214 mm	0.18 - 0.31

OS
Focus: -1.00 dpt Depth: 2.75 mm Operator: --- IOP: ---
Std Dev: 8 µm

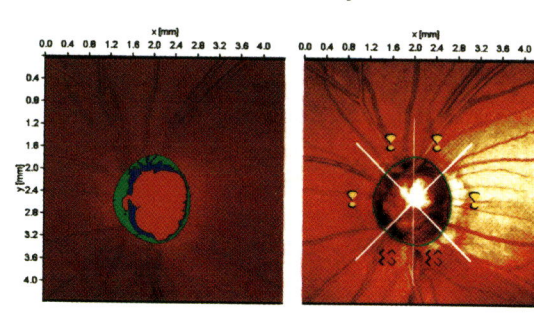

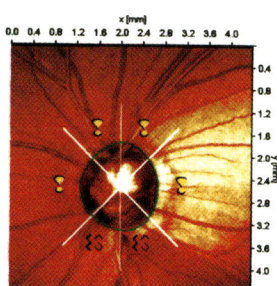

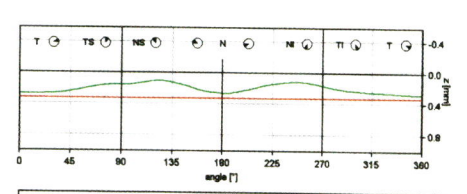

Stereometric Analysis		Normal
Rim Area	0.683 mm²	1.20 - 1.78
Rim Volume	0.092 cmm	0.24 - 0.49
Linear Cup/Disk Ratio	0.775	0.36 - 0.80
Cup Shape Measure	-0.078	-0.27 - -0.09
Height Variation Contour	0.175 mm	0.30 - 0.47
Mean RNFL Thickness	0.124 mm	0.18 - 0.31

OU - Current Exam
- OD contour line
- OS contour line

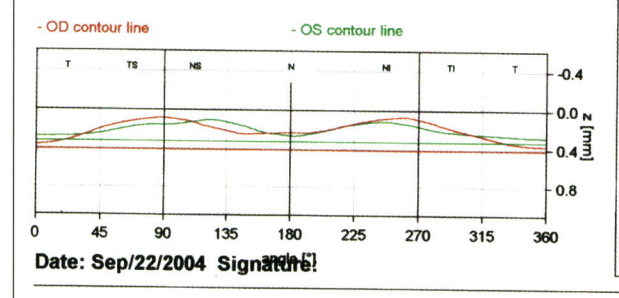

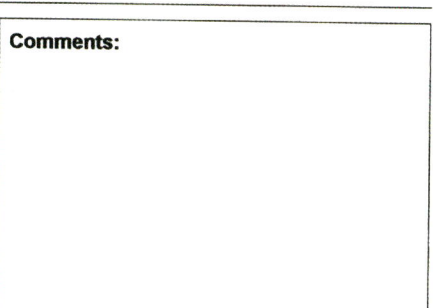

Comments:

Date: Sep/22/2004 Signature:

Software: IR1-V1.7/900

GLAUCOMA PROGRESSION

1. Part of a nine-year follow-up the right eye of a patient with open-angle glaucoma. Reflectivity images (A), topography images (B), reflectivity images with the probability symbols from the Topographic Change Analysis program of the Heidelberg Eye Explorer (C) and grey scale printout from the 30-2 program of the Humphrey Field Analyzer (D). The patient shows a clear change initially in the superior temporal rim with a nerve fiber layer defect and the subsequent collapse of the whole temporal rim. The visual field shows concomitant change with the development of a dense paracentral scotoma.

   (Case was reproduced with kind permission from Dr. B. Chauhan.)

HRT II Primer Cases | FINGERET 109

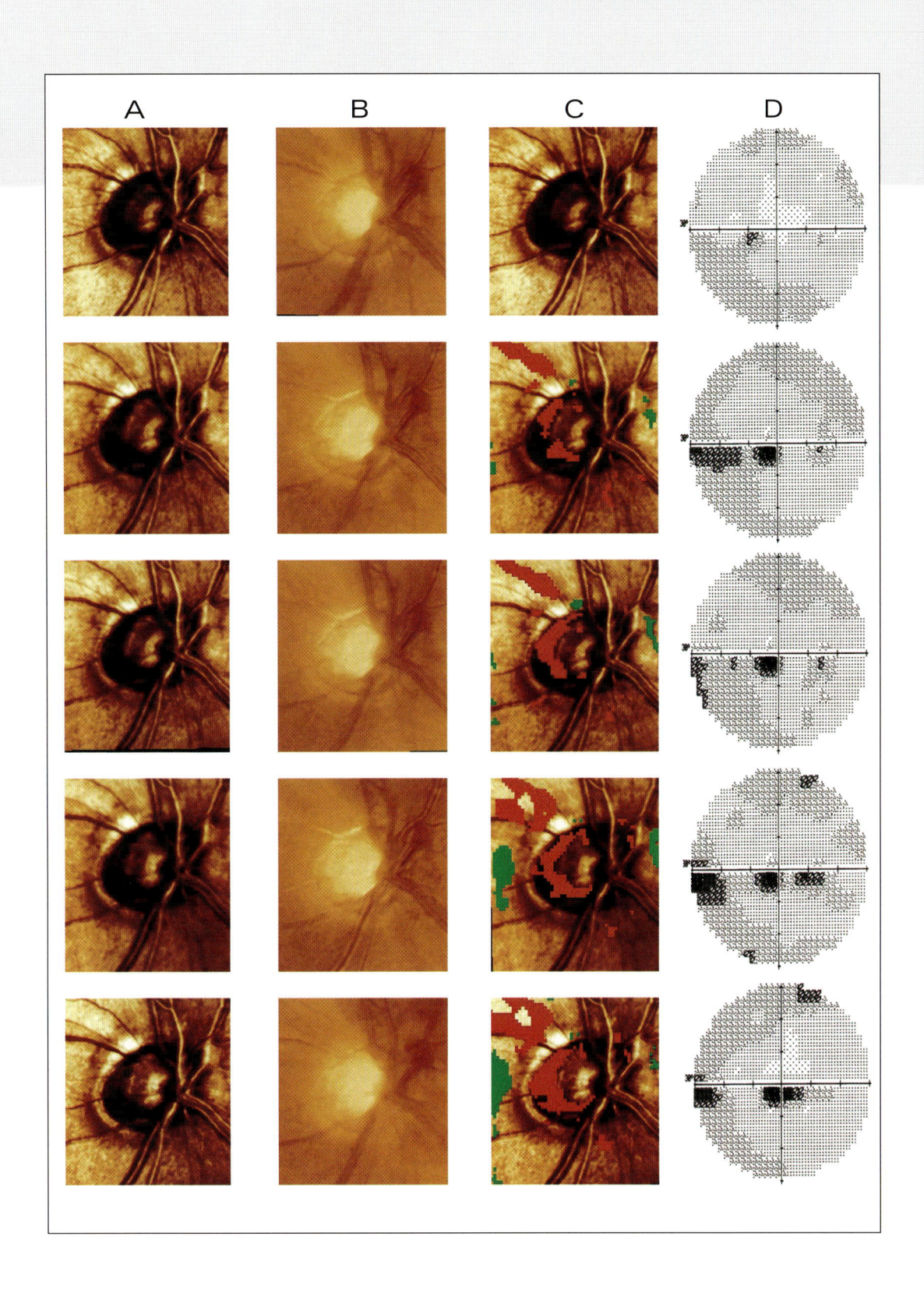

2. This case is of a 69-year-old black male with POAG who has been followed for over 10 years. His IOPs are 14–16 mm Hg, but his central corneal thickness is 470 µm OU. The patient has a history of diabetic retinopathy with laser photocoagulation. He is currently being treated with Travatan OU qhs. The fundus photographs show a vertically elongated cup with rim thinning superiorly and inferiorly, worse superiorly OU. Rim thinning is greater OS than OD. Standard automated white-on-white visual fields reveal an inferior arcuate scotoma OU. The Glaucoma Progression Analysis (GPA) OD shows a cluster of contiguous points in the inferior region with a significant change at the $p < 5\%$ level on two consecutive tests. This is indicative of a worsening visual field. For OS, the GPA reveals only one point at this significance level and is not indicative of a progressing visual field. The HRT results are shown in the OU follow-up printout, the computer screen display of the progression analysis, and the trend analysis. For the right eye, the printout shows progressive enlargement of the cup in the superior region as indicated by the cluster of red superpixels in the Change Probability Map. This superior damage corresponds with the progressing inferior visual field defect as detected by the GPA. In contrast, for OS, the Change Probability Map shows no large clusters of red or green superpixels, indicating no significant structural changes. This also agrees with the stable visual fields. The analysis displayed on the computer screen shows the topography maps on the first row, the reflectance images with the change analysis superimposed on the second row, and the difference maps on the bottom row. The baseline exam is on the leftmost column and each successive follow-up is to the right of the baseline image. Each follow-up is compared to the baseline exam and if the change is statistically significant and present in the same location on two to three consecutive follow-ups, the change will be highlighted as red (for a decrease in height indicating progression) or green (for an increase in height likely due to a remodeling of the retinal surface which often accompanies progression). For OD the damage is progressing superiorly, and for OS the eye is relatively stable. The trend analysis for OD shows a decrease in rim area for the temporal superior and temporal inferior regions (note the overall rim area decreases very little, indicating a worsening of focal damage).

HRT II Primer Cases | FINGERET 111

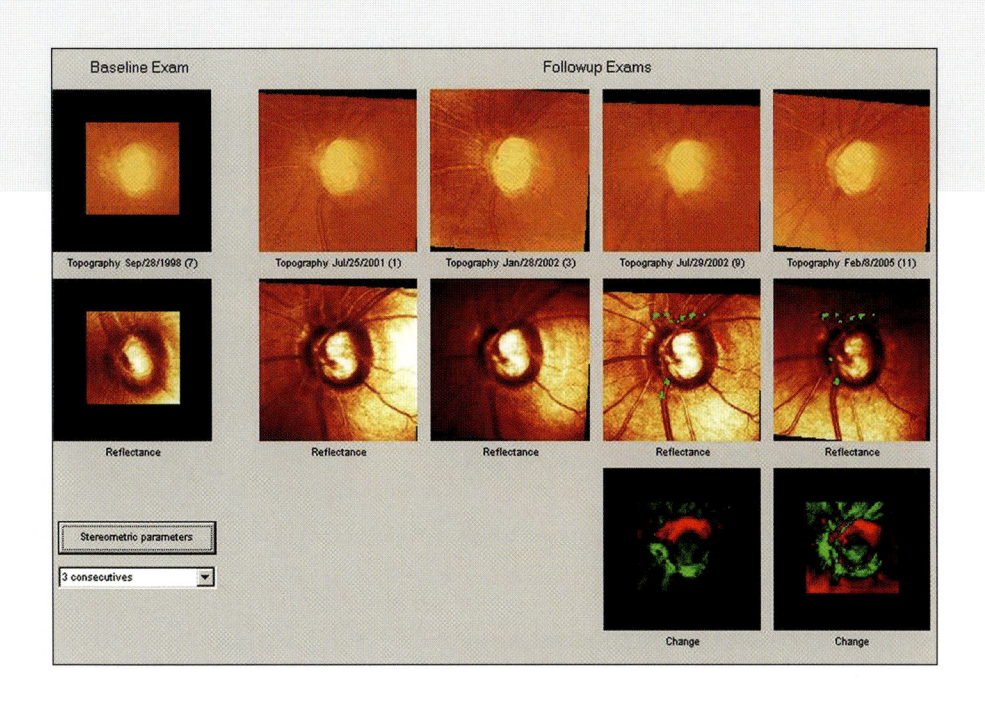

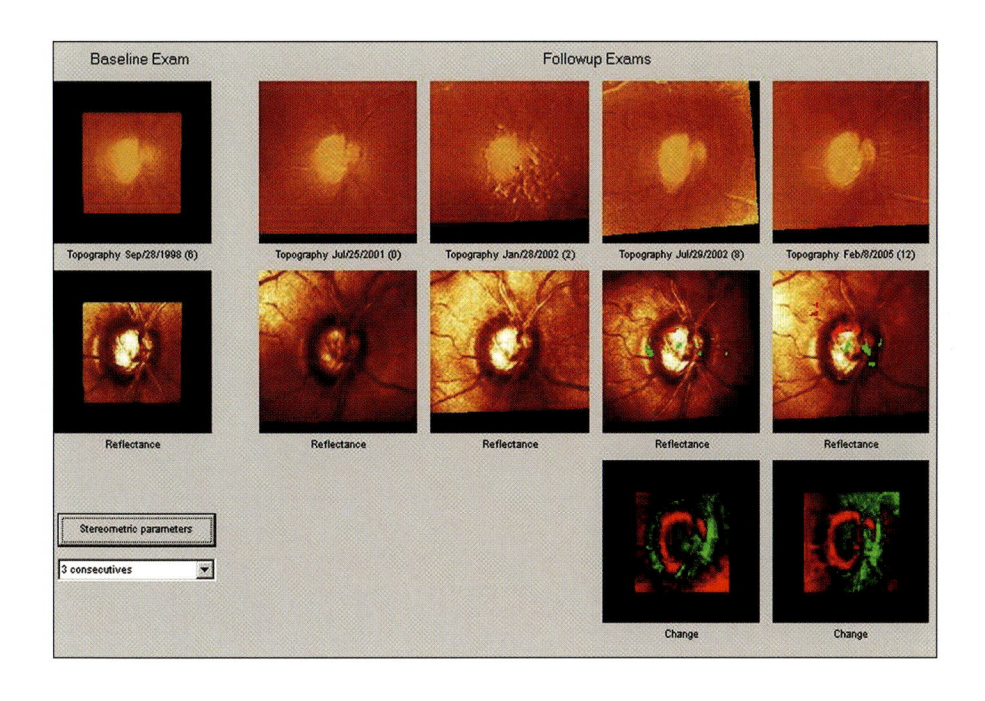

Comments:
OD disc size 2.649
linear c/d 0.703

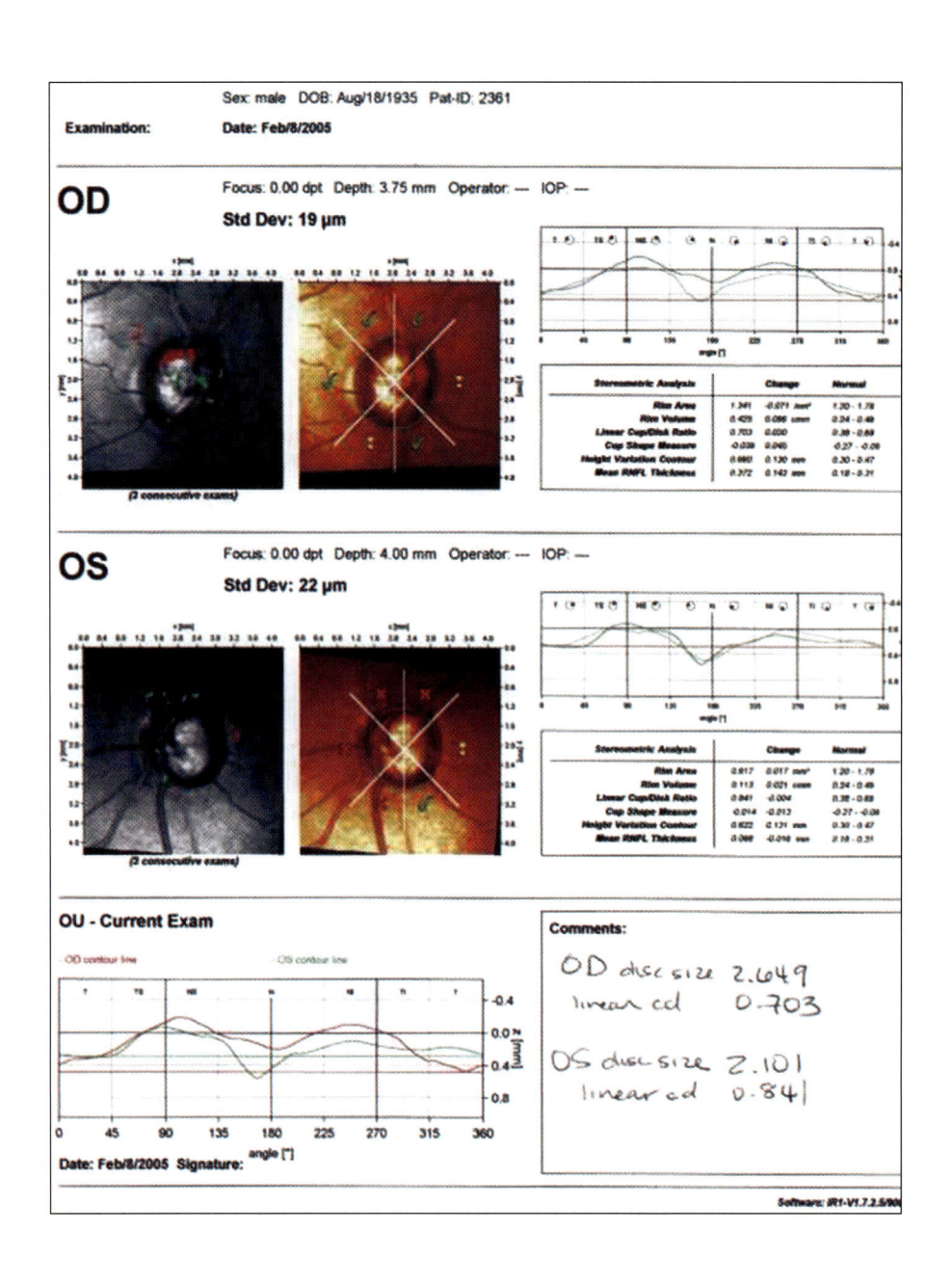

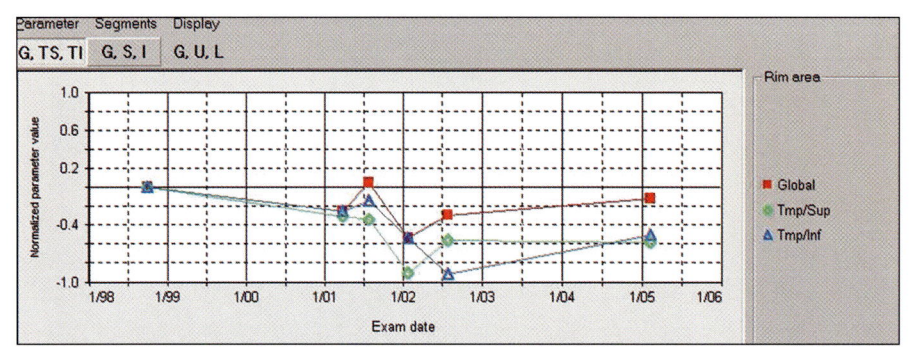

OS disc size 2.101
linear c/d 0.841

112 FINGERET | HRT II Primer Cases

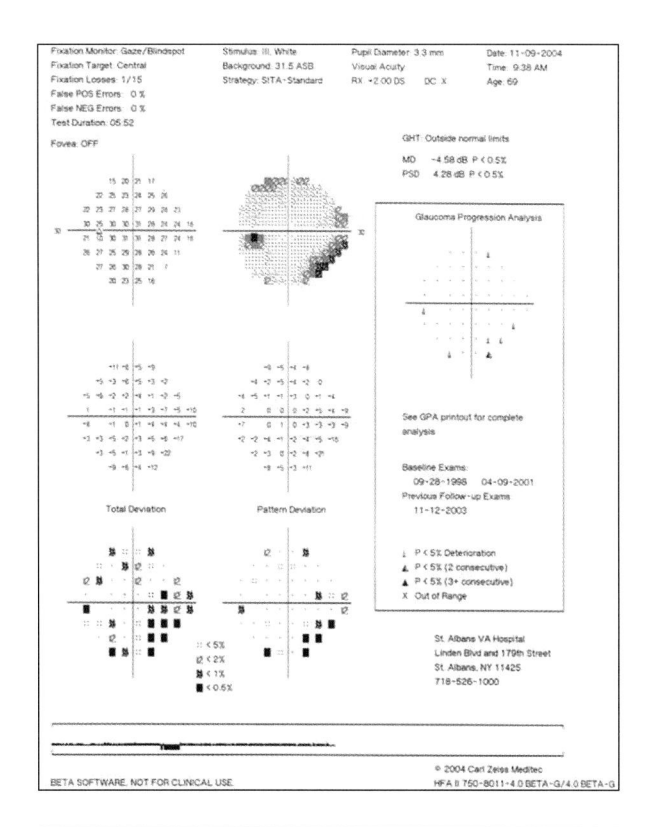

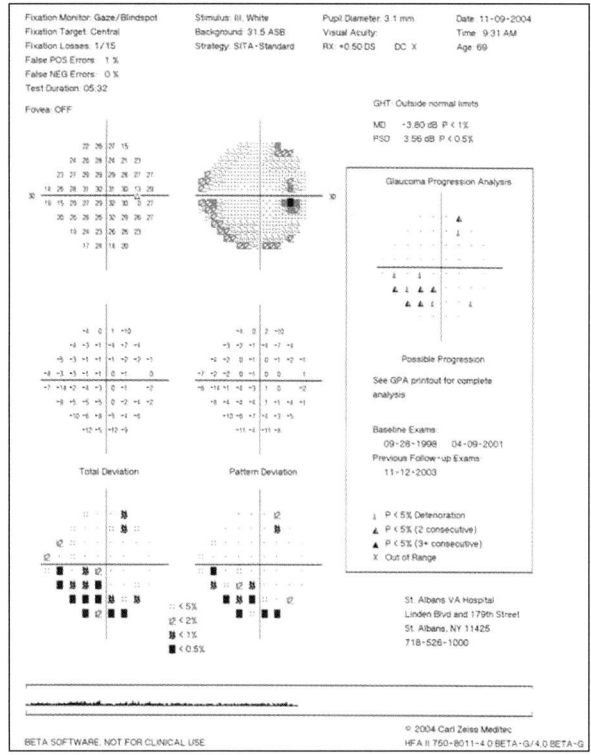

RETINA EDEMA

1. This case illustrates clinically significant diabetic macular edema in a 55-year-old male with type 2 diabetes mellitus of 17 years duration. Late-phase fluorescein angiography (FA) showed pooling in the macular region of the left eye (panel 2). Best corrected visual acuity was 20/15 (OS). Baseline HRT Edema Maps were consistent with the FA and demonstrated a central zone edema index (EI) of 1.60 au. Note that the reflectivity image was used to center the 9-Zone grid on the fovea (panels 3 and 4). Ten weeks later the EI was 2.37 au (panel 5) and 22 weeks later it had increased to 3.62 au. Best corrected visual acuity at the last visit was 20/20-1.

   (Case was reproduced with kind permission from Dr. C. Hudson, Dr. K. Guan, Dr. J. Flanagan, and the Retinal Service of the Toronto Western Hospital.)

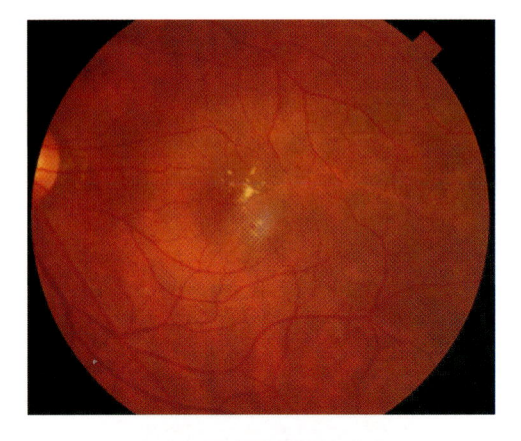

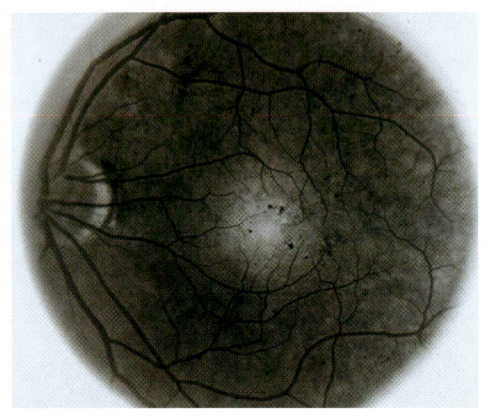

HRT II Primer Cases | FINGERET 115

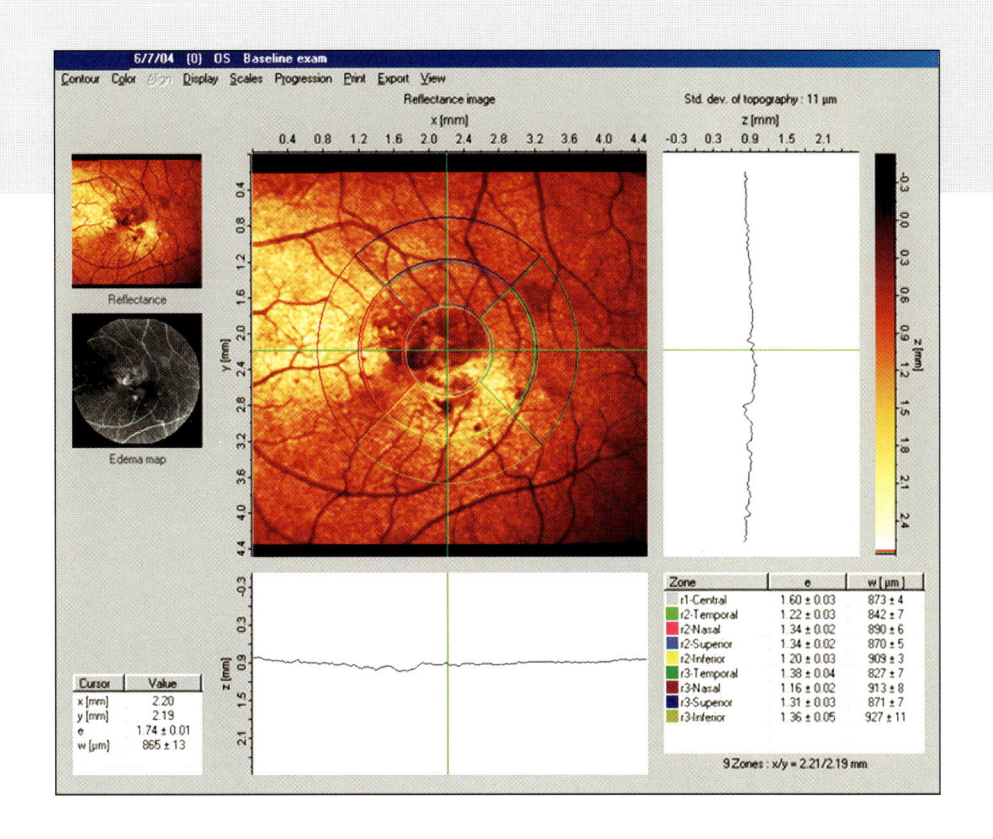

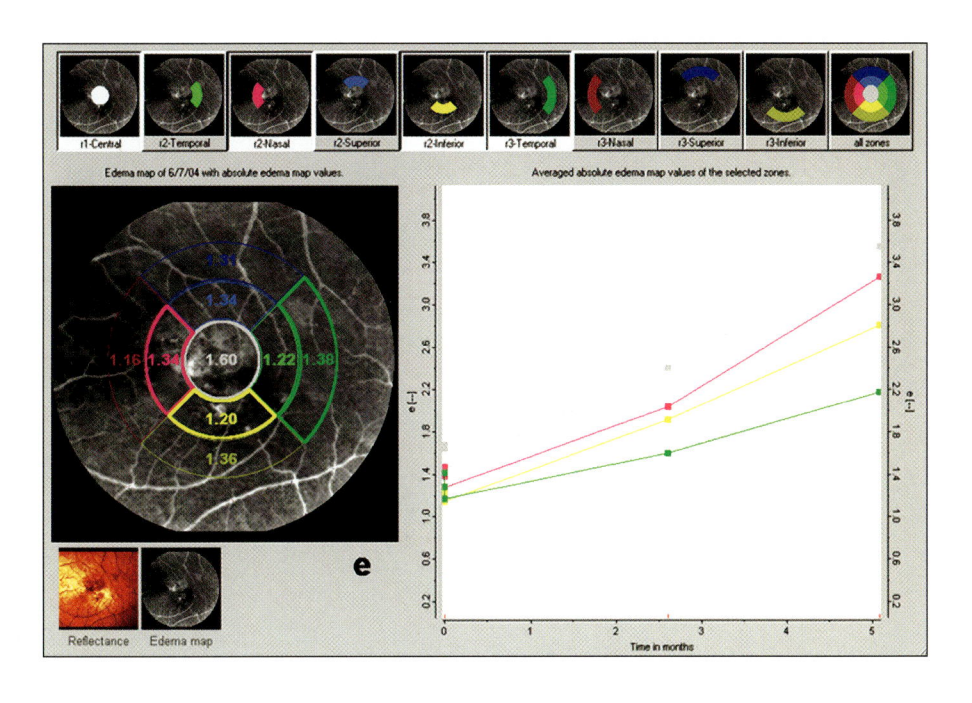

116 FINGERET | HRT II Primer Cases

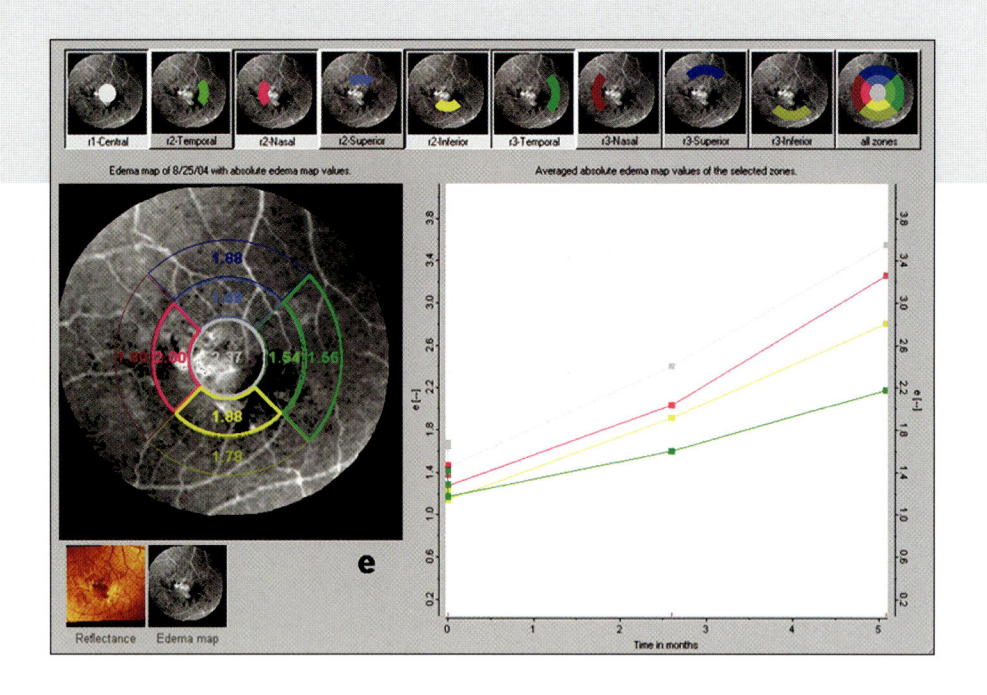

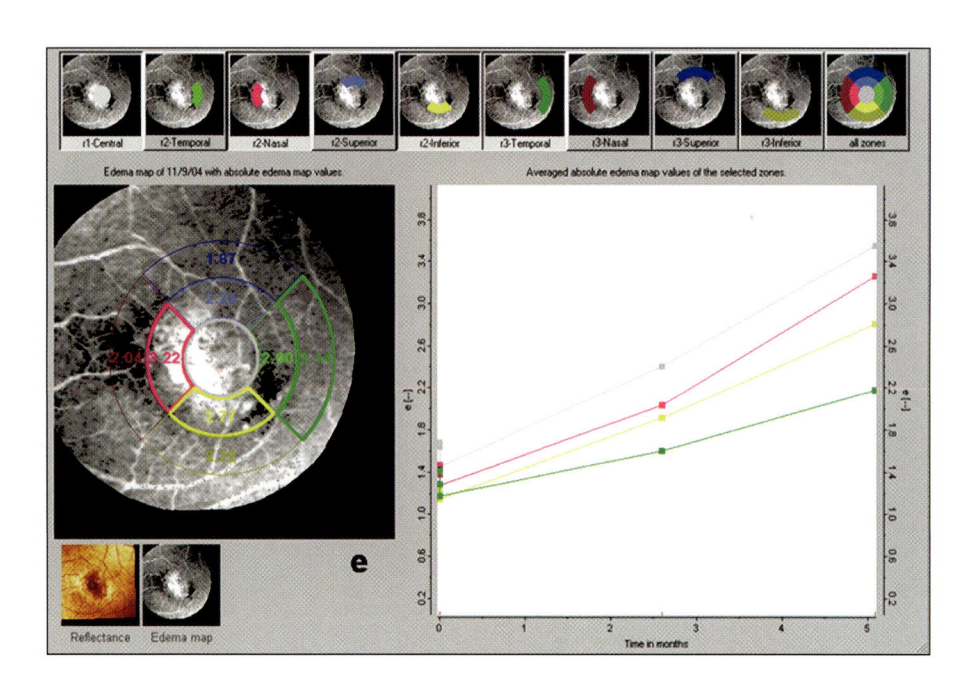

2. A fifty-five-year old male presented complaining of blurred vision in the right eye for three weeks. Best corrected visual acuity was OD 20/200 and OS 20/25. Slit-lamp examination revealed a macular neurosensory retinal detachment in the right eye (panel 1). Fluorescein angiography (FA) demonstrated a focal retinal pigment epithelium leakage consistent with central serous retinopathy (panel 2). HRT Edema Maps showed fluid in the retina with a central zone edema index of 1.89 au OD (panel 3). The same zone for the left eye was 0.87 au. Ten weeks later the central zone gave an edema index of 0.79 au (panels 4 and 5) and visual acuity had improved to 20/40. FA was not repeated.

(Case was reproduced with kind permission from Dr. M. Fromer.)

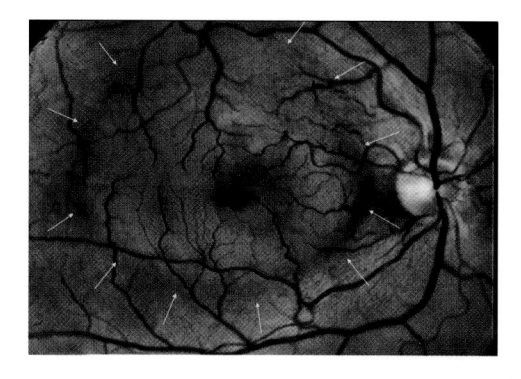

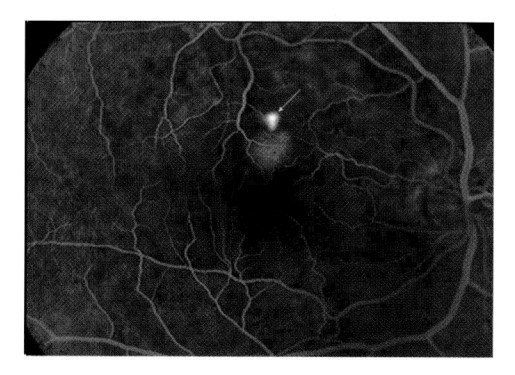

118 FINGERET | HRT II Primer Cases

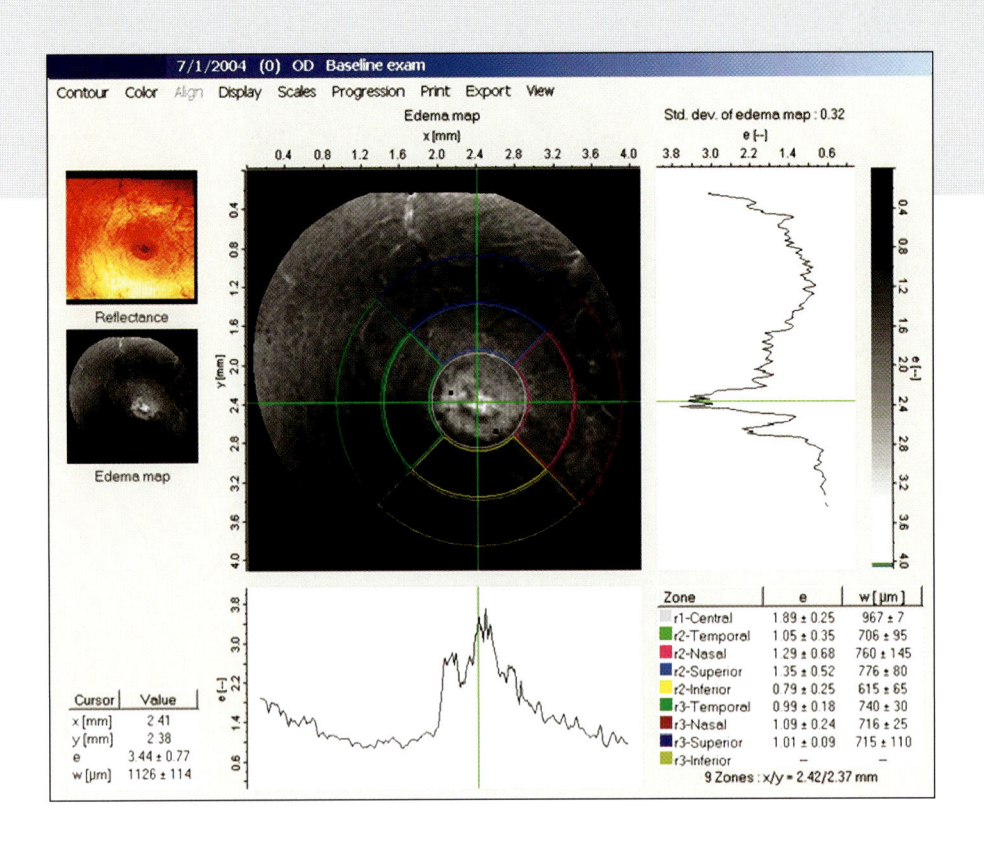

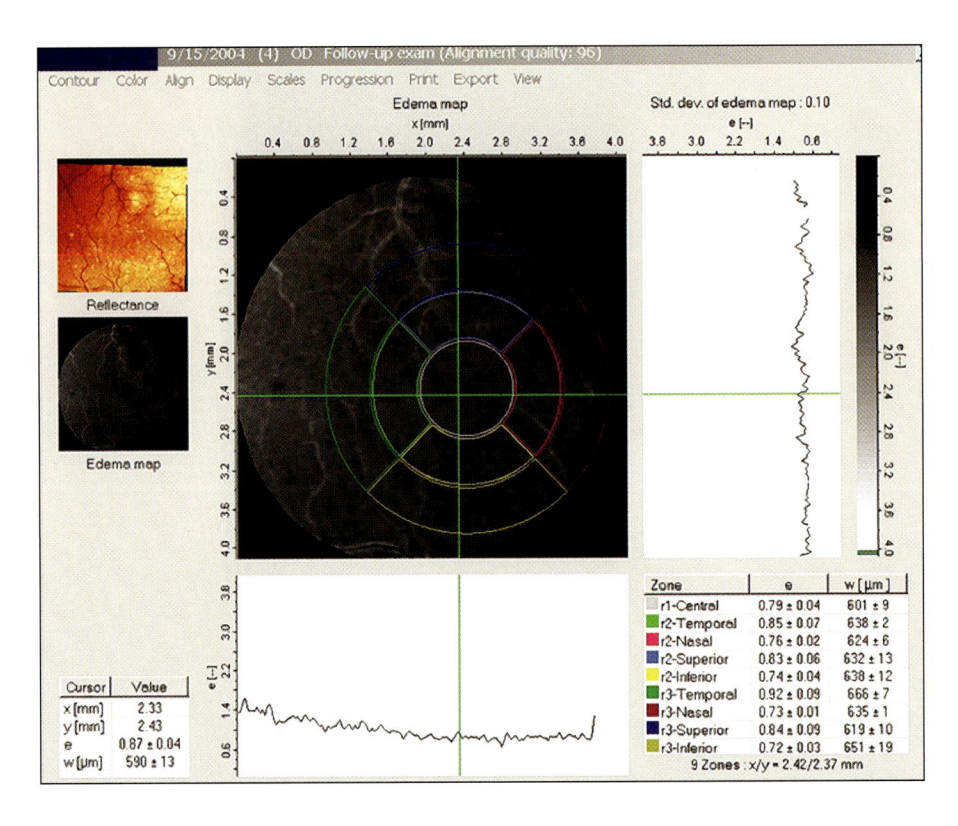

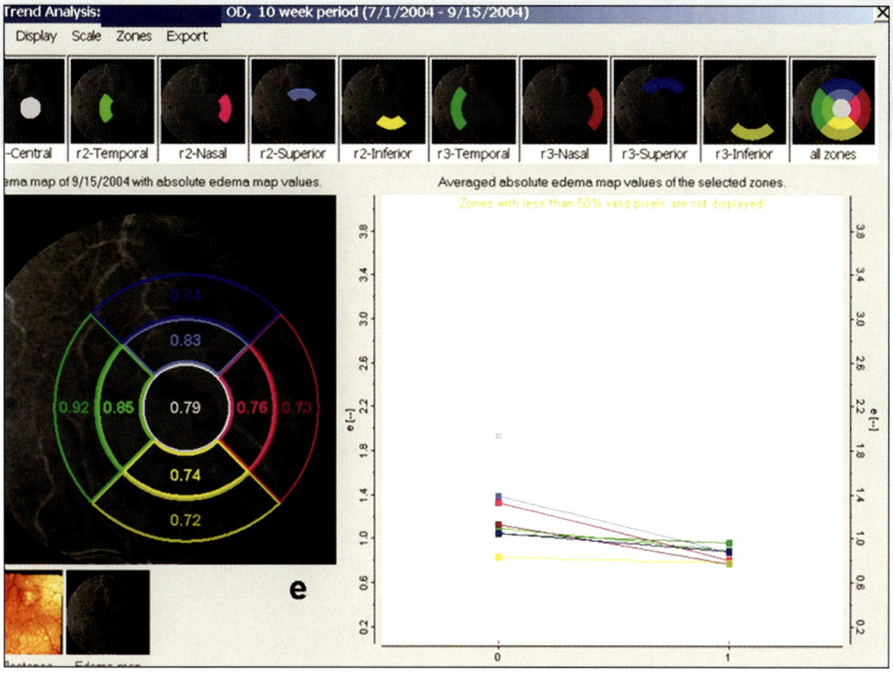
Trend Analysis:
OD, 10 week period (7/1/2004 - 9/15/2004)
Display Scale Zones Export
-Central
r2-Temporal
r2-Nasal
r2-Superior
r2-Inferior
r3-Temporal
r3-Nasal
r3-Superior
r3-Inferior
all zones
ema map of 9/15/2004 with absolute edema map values.
Averaged absolute edema map values of the selected zones.
0.83
0.92
0.85
0.79
0.76
0.74
0.72
e
e [-]

SUGGESTED READINGS

GLAUCOMA

Ocular Hypertension Treatment Study (OHTS) Ancillary Study

Zangwill LM, Weinreb RN, Beiser JA, et al. Baseline topographic optic disc measurements are associated with the development of primary open angle glaucoma: the Confocal Scanning Laser Ophthalmoscopy Ancillary Study to the Ocular Hypertension Treatment Study. *Arch Ophthalmol*. 2005 (in press).

Zangwill LM, Weinreb RN, Berry CC, et al. The confocal scanning laser ophthalmoscopy ancillary study to the ocular hypertension treatment study: study design and baseline factors. *Am J Ophthalmol*. 2004;137:219-227.

Zangwill LM, Weinreb RN, Berry CC, et al. Racial differences in optic disc topography: baseline results from the confocal scanning laser ophthalmoscopy ancillary study to the ocular hypertension treatment study. *Arch Ophthalmol*. 2004;122:22-28.

Comparison with optic disc photography

Wollstein G, Garway-Heath DF, Fontana L, Hitchings RA. Identifying early glaucomatous changes. Comparison between expert clinical assessment of optic disc photographs and confocal scanning ophthalmoscopy. *Ophthalmology*. 2000;107:2272-2277.

Zangwill L, Shakiba S, Caprioli J, Weinreb RN. Agreement between clinicians and a confocal scanning laser ophthalmoscope in estimating cup/disk ratios. *Am J Ophthalmol*. 1995;119:415-421.

Diagnostic accuracy (cross-sectional studies)

Chen E. Ratio of hemi-papillary rim volumes and glaucoma diagnosis with Heidelberg retina tomograph. *J Glaucoma*. 2005;14:206-209.

Zangwill LM, Chan K, Bowd C, et al. Heidelberg retina tomograph measurements of the optic disc and parapapillary retina for detecting glaucoma analyzed by machine learning classifiers. *Invest Ophthalmol Vis Sci*. 2004;45:3144-3151.

Medeiros FA, Zangwill LM, Bowd C, Weinreb RN. Comparison of the GDx VCC scanning laser polarimeter, HRT II confocal scanning laser ophthalmoscope, and Stratus OCT optical coherence tomograph for the detection of glaucoma. *Arch Ophthalmol*. 2004;122:827-837.

Miglior S, Guareschi M, Albe' E, Gomarasca S, Vavassori M, Orzalesi N. Detection of glaucomatous visual field changes using the Moorfields regression analysis of the Heidelberg retina tomograph. *Am J Ophthalmol*. 2003;136:26-33.

Kiriyama N, Ando A, Fukui C, et al. A comparison of optic disc topographic parameters in patients with primary open angle glaucoma, normal tension glaucoma, and ocular hypertension. *Graefes Arch Clin Exp Ophthalmol*. 2003;241:541-545.

Bowd C, Chan K, Zangwill LM, et al. Comparing neural networks and linear discriminant functions for glaucoma detection using confocal scanning laser ophthalmoscopy of the optic disc. *Invest Ophthalmol Vis Sci*. 2002;43:3444-3454.

Zangwill LM, Bowd C, Berry CC, et al. Discriminating between normal and glaucomatous eyes using the Heidelberg Retina Tomograph, GDx Nerve Fiber Analyzer, and Optical Coherence Tomograph. *Arch Ophthalmol*. 2001;119:985-993.

Swindale NV, Stjepanovic G, Chin A, Mikelberg FS. Automated analysis of normal and glaucomatous optic nerve head topography images. *Invest Ophthalmol Vis Sci*. 2000; 41:1730-1742.

Wollstein G, Garway-Heath DF, Poinoosawmy D, Hitchings RA. Glaucomatous optic disc changes in the contralateral eye of unilateral normal pressure glaucoma patients. *Ophthalmology*. 2000;107:2267-2271.

Mardin CY, Horn FK, Jonas JB, Budde WM. Preperimetric glaucoma diagnosis by confocal scanning laser tomography of the optic disc. *Br J Ophthalmol*. 1999;83:299-304.

Wollstein G, Garway-Heath DF, Hitchings RA. Identification of early glaucoma cases with the scanning laser ophthalmoscope. *Ophthalmology*. 1998;105:1557-1563.

Iester M, Mikelberg FS, Drance SM. The effect of optic disc size on diagnostic precision with the Heidelberg Retina Tomograph. *Ophthalmology*. 1997;104:545-548.

Uchida H, Brigatti L, Caprioli J. Detection of structural damage from glaucoma with confocal laser image analysis. *Invest Ophthalmol Vis Sci*. 1996;37:2393-2401.

Histology correlation

Yucel YH, Gupta N, Kalichman MW, et al. Relationship of optic disc topography to optic nerve fiber number in glaucoma. *Arch Ophthalmol*. 1998;116:493-497.

Screening

Robin TA, Muller A, Rait J, Keeffe JE, Taylor HR, Mukesh BN. Performance of community-based glaucoma screening using frequency doubling technology and Heidelberg retinal tomography. *Ophthalmic Epidemiol*. 2005;12:167-178.

Sponsel WE. Integrating numerical indices of structure and function to optimize diagnostic sensitivity and specificity in screening for glaucoma. *Ophthalmic Epidemiol*. 2005;12:163-166.

Nonglaucomatous neuropathies

Danesh-Meyer H, Savino PJ, Spaeth GL, Gamble GD. Comparison of arteritis and nonarteritic anterior ischemic optic neuropathies with the Heidelberg Retina Tomograph. *Ophthalmology*. 2005;112:1104-1112.

Plummer DJ, Bartsch DU, Azen SP, Max S, Sadun AA, Freeman WR. Retinal nerve fiber layer evaluation in human immunodeficiency virus-positive patients. *Am J Ophthalmol*. 2001;131:216-222.

Early detection (longitudinal studies)

Bowd C, Zangwill LM, Medeiros FA, et al. Confocal scanning laser ophthalmoscopy classifiers and stereophotograph evaluation for prediction of visual field abnormalities in glaucoma-suspect eyes. *Invest Ophthalmol Vis Sci*. 2004;45:2255-2262.

Tan JC, Hitchings RA. Optimizing and validating an approach for identifying glaucomatous change in optic nerve topography. *Invest Ophthalmol Vis Sci*. 2004;45:1396-1403.

Tan JC, Poinoosawmy D, Hitchings RA. Tomographic identification of neuroretinal rim loss in high-pressure, normal-pressure, and suspected glaucoma. *Invest Ophthalmol Vis Sci*. 2004;45:2279-2285.

Bathija R, Zangwill L, Berry CC, Sample PA, Weinreb RN. Detection of early glaucomatous structural damage with confocal scanning laser tomography. *J Glaucoma*. 1998;7:121-127.

Progression

Patterson AJ, Garway-Heath DF, Strouthidis NG, Crabb DP. A new statistical approach for quantifying change in series of retinal and optic nerve head topography images. *Invest Ophthalmol Vis Sci*. 2005;46:1659-1667.

Artes PH, Chauhan BC. Longitudinal changes in the visual field and optic disc in glaucoma. *Prog Retin Eye Res*. 2005;24:333-354.

Nicolela MT, McCormick TA, Drance SM, Ferrier SN, LeBlanc RP, Chauhan BC. Visual field and optic disc progression in patients with different types of optic disc damage: a longitudinal prospective study. *Ophthalmology*. 2003;110:2178-2184.

Chauhan BC, McCormick TA, Nicolela MT, LeBlanc RP. Optic disc and visual field changes in a prospective longitudinal study of patients with glaucoma: comparison of scanning laser tomography with conventional perimetry and optic disc photography. *Arch Ophthalmol*. 2001;119:1492-1499.

Chauhan BC, Blanchard JW, Hamilton DC, LeBlanc RP. Technique for detecting serial topographic changes in the optic disc and peripapillary retina using scanning laser tomography. *Invest Ophthalmol Vis Sci*. 2000;41:775-782.

Kamal DS, Garway-Heath DF, Hitchings RA, Fitzke FW. Use of sequential Heidelberg retina tomograph images to identify changes at the optic disc in ocular hypertensive patients at risk of developing glaucoma. *Br J Ophthalmol*. 2000;84:993-998.

Kamal DS, Viswanathan AC, Garway-Heath DF, Hitchings RA, Poinoosawmy D, Bunce C. Detection of optic disc change with the Heidelberg retina tomograph before confirmed visual field change in ocular hypertensives converting to early glaucoma. *Br J Ophthalmol.* 1999;83:290-294.

Reproducibility

Miglior S, Albe E, Guareschi M, Rossetti L, Orzalesi N. Intraobserver and interobserver reproducibility in the evaluation of optic disc stereometric parameters by Heidelberg Retina Tomograph. *Ophthalmology.* 2002;109:1072-1077.

Hatch WV, Flanagan JG, Williams-Lyn DE, Buys YM, Farra T, Trope GE. Interobserver agreement of Heidelberg retina tomograph parameters. *J Glaucoma.* 1999;8:232-237.

Bathija R, Zangwill L, Berry CC, Sample PA, Weinreb RN. Detection of early glaucomatous structural damage with confocal scanning laser tomography. *J Glaucoma.* 1998;7:121-127.

Caprioli J, Park HJ, Ugurlu S, Hoffman D. Slope of the peripapillary nerve fiber layer surface in glaucoma. *Invest Ophthalmol Vis Sci.* 1998;39:2321-2328.

Tomita G, Honbe K, Kitazawa Y. Reproducibility of measurements by laser scanning tomography in eyes before and after pilocarpine treatment. *Graefes Arch Clin Exp Ophthalmol.* 1994;232:406-408.

Chauhan BC, LeBlanc RP, McCormick TA, Rogers JB. Test-retest variability of topographic measurements with confocal scanning laser tomography in patients with glaucoma and control subjects. *Am J Ophthalmol.* 1994;118:9-15.

Rohrschneider K, Burk RO, Kruse FE, Volcker HE. Reproducibility of the optic nerve head topography with a new laser tomographic scanning device. *Ophthalmology.* 1994;101:1044-1049.

Weinreb RN, Lusky M, Bartsch DU, Morsman D. Effect of repetitive imaging on topographic measurements of the optic nerve head. *Arch Ophthalmol.* 1993;111:636-638.

Correlation with visual fields

Greenstein VC, Thienprasiddhi P, Ritch R, Liebmann JM, Hood DC. A method for comparing electrophysiological, psychophysical, and structural measures of glaucomatous damage. *Arch Ophthalmol.* 2004;122:1276-1284.

Bosworth CF, Sample PA, Williams JM, Zangwill L, Lee B, Weinreb RN. Spatial relationship of motion automated perimetry and optic disc topography in patients with glaucomatous optic neuropathy. *J Glaucoma.* 1999;8:281-289.

Iester M, Courtright P, Mikelberg FS. Retinal nerve fiber layer height in high-tension glaucoma and healthy eyes [published erratum appears in *J Glaucoma* 1998;7:296]. *J Glaucoma.* 1998;7:1-7.

Anton A, Yamagishi N, Zangwill L, Sample PA, Weinreb RN. Mapping structural to functional damage in glaucoma with standard automated perimetry and confocal scanning laser ophthalmoscopy. *Am J Ophthalmol.* 1998;125:436-446.

Teesalu P, Vihanninjoki K, Airaksinen PJ, Tuulonen A. Hemifield association between blue-on-yellow visual field and optic nerve head topographic measurements. *Graefes Arch Clin Exp Ophthalmol.* 1998;236:339-345.

Iester M, Mikelberg FS, Courtright P, Drance SM. Correlation between the visual field indices and Heidelberg retina tomograph parameters. *J Glaucoma.* 1997;6:78-82.

Teesalu P, Vihanninjoki K, Airaksinen PJ, Tuulonen A, Läärä E. Correlation of blue-on-yellow visual fields with scanning confocal laser optic disc measurements. *Invest Ophthalmol Vis Sci.* 1997;38:2452-2459.

Iester M, Swindale NV, Mikelberg FS. Sector-based analysis of optic nerve head shape parameters and visual field indices in healthy and glaucomatous eyes. *J Glaucoma.* 1997;6:370-376.

Brigatti L, Caprioli J. Correlation of visual field with scanning confocal laser optic disc measurements in glaucoma [published erratum appears in Arch Ophthalmol 1996;114:424]. *Arch Ophthalmol.* 1995;113:1191-1194.

Miscellaneous

Vernon SA, Hawker MJ, Ainsworth G, Hillman JG, Macnab HK, Dua HS. Laser scanning tomography of the optic nerve head in a normal elderly population: the Bridlington Eye Assessment Project. *Invest Ophthalmol Vis Sci.* 2005;46:2823-2828.

Iester M, Mermoud A. Retinal nerve fiber layer measured by Heidelberg retina tomograph and nerve fiber analyzer. *Eur J Ophthalmol.* 2005;15:246-254.

Harasymowycz P, Davis B, Xu G, Myers J, Bayer A, Spaeth GL. The use of RADAAR (ratio of rim area to disc area asymmetry) in detecting glaucoma and its severity. *Can J Ophthalmol.* 2004;39:240-244.

Ahn JK, Park KH. Morphometric change analysis of the optic nerve head in unilateral disk hemorrhage cases. *Am J Ophthalmol.* 2002;134:920-922.

Bowd C, Weinreb RN, Lee B, Emdadi A, Zangwill LM. Optic disk topography after medical treatment to reduce intraocular pressure. *Am J Ophthalmol.* 2000;130:280-286.

Zangwill LM, Berry CC, Weinreb RN. Optic disc topographic measurements after pupil dilation. *Ophthalmology.* 1999;106:1751-1755.

Topouzis F, Peng F, Kotas-Neumann R, et al. Longitudinal changes in optic disc topography of adult patients after trabeculectomy. *Ophthalmology.* 1999;106:1147-1151.

Burk RO, Tuulonen A, Airaksinen PJ. Laser scanning tomography of localised nerve fibre layer defects. *Br J Ophthalmol.* 1998;82:1112-1117.

Emdadi A, Zangwill L, Sample PA, Kono Y, Anton A, Weinreb RN. Patterns of optic disk damage in patients with early focal visual field loss. *Am J Ophthalmol.* 1998;126:763-771.

Irak I, Zangwill L, Garden V, Shakiba S, Weinreb RN. Change in optic disk topography after trabeculectomy. *Am J Ophthalmol*. 1996;122:690-695.

RETINA

Detection of maculopathy

Bishop F, Walters G, Geall M, Woon H. Scanning laser tomography of full thickness idiopathic macular holes. *Eye*. 2005;19:123-128.

Guan K, Hudson C, Flanagan JG. Comparison of Heidelberg Retina Tomograph II and Retinal Thickness Analyzer in the assessment of diabetic macular edema. *Invest Ophthalmol Vis Sci*. 2004;45:610-616.

Bartsch DU, Aurora A, Rodanant N, Cheng L, Freeman WR. Volumetric analysis of macular edema by scanning laser tomography in immune recovery uveitis. *Arch Ophthalmol*. 2003;121:1246-1251.

Tong L, Ang A, Vernon SA, et al. Sensitivity and specificity of a new scoring system for diabetic macular oedema detection using a confocal laser imaging system. *Br J Ophthalmol*. 2001;85:34-39.

Kobayashi H, Kobayashi K. Quantitative measurements of changes of idiopathic stage 3 macular holes after vitrectomy using confocal scanning laser tomography. *Graefes Arch Clin Exp Ophthalmol*. 2000;238:410-419.

Akiba J, Yanagiya N, Konno S, Hikichi T, Yoshida A. Three-dimensional characteristics of macular pseudoholes using confocal laser tomography. *Ophthalmic Surg Lasers*. 1999;30:513-517.

Jaakkola A, Vesti E, Immonen I. The use of confocal scanning laser tomography in the evaluation of retinal elevation in age-related macular degeneration. *Ophthalmology*. 1999;106:274-279.

Hudson C, Charles SJ, Flanagan JG, Brahma AK, Turner GS, McLeod D. Objective morphological assessment of macular hole surgery by scanning laser tomography. *Br J Ophthalmol*. 1997;81:107-116.

Weinberger D, Stiebel H, Gaton DD, Friedland S, Priel E, Yassur Y. Three-dimensional measurements of central serous chorioretinopathy using a scanning laser tomograph. *Am J Ophthalmol*. 1996;122:864-869.

Weinberger D, Stiebel H, Gaton DD, Priel E, Yassur Y. Three-dimensional measurements of idiopathic macular holes using a scanning laser tomograph. *Ophthalmology*. 1995;102:1445-1449.

Reproducibility

Pallikaris A, Skondra D, Tsilimbaris M. Intraobserver repeatability of macula measurements by confocal scanning laser tomography. *Am J Ophthalmol*. 2005;139:624-630.

Ang A, Tong L, Vernon SA. Improvement of reproducibility of macular volume measurements using the Heidelberg retinal tomograph. *Br J Ophthalmol*. 2000;84:1194-1197.

Zambarakji HJ, Amoaku WM, Vernon SA. Volumetric analysis of early macular edema with the Heidelberg Retina Tomograph in diabetic retinopathy. *Ophthalmology*. 1998;105:1051-1059.

Zambarakji HJ, Evans JE, Amoaku WM, Vernon SA. Reproducibility of volumetric measurements of normal maculae with the Heidelberg retina tomograph. *Br J Ophthalmol*. 1998;82:884-891.

Menezes AV, Giunta M, Chisholm L, Harvey PT, Tuli R, Devenyi RG. Reproducibility of topographic measurements of the macula with a scanning laser ophthalmoscope. *Ophthalmology*. 1995;102:230-235.

Technology

Hudson C, Flanagan JG, Turner GS, McLeod D. Scanning laser tomography Z profile signal width as an objective index of macular retinal thickening. *Br J Ophthalmol*. 1998;82:121-130.

Correlation with visual function

Hudson C, Flanagan JG, Turner GS, Chen HC, Young LB, McLeod D. Correlation of a scanning laser derived oedema index and visual function following grid laser treatment for diabetic macular oedema. *Br J Ophthalmol*. 2003;87:455-461.

Kobayashi H, Kobayashi K. Correlation of quantitative three-dimensional measurements of macular hole size with visual acuity after vitrectomy. *Graefes Arch Clin Exp Ophthalmol*. 1999;237:283-288.